Aging and Dementia

Mechteld van Kooi MSc is gratefully acknowledged for her critical reading and excellent editing of the manuscript and publisher Jan Oegema PhD for his enthousiastic coaching of the project.

VU University Press
De Boelelaan 1105
1081 HV Amsterdam
The Netherlands

info@vu-uitgeverij.nl
www.vuuitgeverij.nl

© 2011 by the author

Design cover: Communications Department VU (Heleen ten Voorde)
Photo front cover: Jan Oegema
Photo back cover: Communications Department VU (Riechelle van der Valk)
Type setting: JAPES, Amsterdam (Jaap Prummel)

ISBN 978 90 8659 561 7
NUR 770, 870

Aging and Dementia

Neuropsychology, Motor Skills, and Pain

Erik Scherder

VU University Press
Amsterdam

Table of Contents

Chapter 1
Epidemiology and neuropathology in aging and dementia

1.1 Introduction

First, epidemiology of aging, Mild Cognitive Impairment (MCI), Alzheimer's disease, vascular dementia, and frontotemporal dementia will be presented. Subsequently, we will briefly describe the cholinergic basal forebrain and related neurotransmitter systems for their role in arousal and their sensitivity for age-related and dementia-related neuropathology. Next, the neuropathology, where appropriate divided into atrophy, reduced metabolism, neuritic plaques, neurofibrillary tangles, neuronal loss, neurotransmitter deficits, and reduced vascularisation, will be discussed with respect to aging, MCI, Alzheimer's disease, vascular dementia, in particular subcortical ischemic vascular dementia (SIVD), and the frontal and temporal variant of FTD.

1.2 Epidemiology of aging, Mild Cognitive Impairment, and the most prevalent subtypes of dementia

1.2.1 Epidemiology of Aging

It has been suggested that aging of the world's population is the most important demographic change of the former century (Riggs, 1996). In particular, the number of 'oldest-old' (older people above 85 years of age) is growing at the fastest rate in developed countries.

In 1900 3 million people were 65 years of age or older in the United States (Brody, 1992). In 1975 and in 1985 this population had increased up to 20 and 25 million people, respectively, a number that parallels the total population of Canada (Brody, 1992). It is predicted that in 2030 21% of the total population of the United States will belong to the population of 65 years and older (Brody, 1992). It is therefore not surprising that also from a scientific point of view, there is a growing interest in this population.

1.2.2 Epidemiology of Mild Cognitive Impairment

In one study, 5% out of 1315 older participants appeared to have Mild Cognitive Impairment (MCI; Manly et al., 2005). Similar results were reported by others, who found MCI in 4.9 – 9.3% out of 1600 subjects (Tognoni et al., 2005). A number of people with MCI develops Alzheimer's disease (Grundman et al., 2004) but this does not hold for every one (Winblad et al., 2004). MCI patients who show a decline in Instrumental Activities of Daily Life (IADL) have a higher chance of developing Alzheimer's disease (Tuokko, Morris, & Ebert, 2005).

Risk factors for MCI include age, low education, and the presence of Apolipoprotein E4 (Manly et al., 2005; Tognoni et al., 2005), a protein that is involved in lipid metabolism (Roses, 1994).

1.2.3 Epidemiology of Alzheimer's disease

Alzheimer's disease is one of the most common causes of dementia in older people (Román, Erkinjuntti, Wallin, Pantoni, & Chui, 2002) and is the fourth cause of death among adults (Keane, 1994). The prevalence of probable Alzheimer's disease increases with age, i.e., 3% of persons between 65 and 74 years of age, 18.7% of older persons between 75 and 84 years of age and even 47.2% of persons of 85 years of age and older (Evans et al., 1989). These results clearly show that age is the main risk factor for Alzheimer's disease. Other risk factors include 1) the presence of Apolipoprotein E4, 2) severe head trauma (Blass, 1993), 3) multiple small head traumas as they are caused by for example boxing (Tariot, 1994), 4) cardiovascular disease (Blass, 1993, Tariot, 1994), 5) family history with Alzheimer's disease and Down's syndrome (Blass, 1993; Tariot, 1994), presence of extrapyramidal signs (Richards, Stern, Marder, Cote, & Mayeux, 1993), hypothyroidism (van Duijn & Hofman, 1992), 6) gender: more women than men suffer from Alzheimer's disease than men (Blass, 1993). Of note is that the prevalence of Alzheimer's disease is inversely related to the level of education, i.e., the higher the level of education, the lower the risk for Alzheimer's disease (Mortimer & Graves, 1993).

'Wear and tear' versus 'use it or lose it'
As suggested before, age is the main risk factor for Alzheimer's disease (Evans et al., 1989; Blass, 1993; Drachman, 1997). The question arises why the aging brain is more sensitive for diseases and why the aging brain is less able to cope with the consequences of diseases (Drachman, 1997). The answer to this question emerges from two theories. The first theory implies that the process of degeneration and death that accompanies aging is genetically programmed, a process called 'apopto-

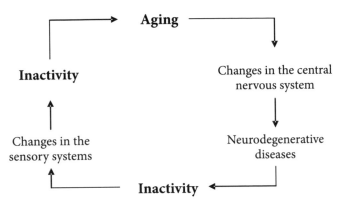

Figure 1. A 'vicious circle of accelerated aging' is indicating that aging coincides with changes in the central nervous system, making the central nervous system more vulnerable for the onset of neurodegenerative diseases, causing inactivity. Inactivity together with age-related accelerated changes in the sensory systems further enhances inactivity and accelerates the aging process.

sis' (Drachman, 1997). The second theory is paraphrased as 'wear and tear' (Swaab, 1991).

'Wear and tear'
During the lifespan, organisms 'wear and tear', because they are continuously active (compare the wearing of a pair of shoes) (Swaab, 1991). The release of free radicals plays an important role in this process (Drachman, 1997; Harman, 1981). Free radicals are produced during aerobic (oxidative) metabolism (Drachman, 1997; Harman, 1981), are most harmful for the organism and contribute to accelerated aging of the cells (Drachman, 1997). Free radicals may also contribute to the neuropathology of Alzheimer's disease (Harman, 1981). Within the scope of free radicals, it appears to be important to avoid overweight from childhood instead of losing weight at an older age (Cohen & Havlik, 1993). Favourable effects of anti-oxidants such as vitamins E and C on certain types of cancer and auto-immune diseases have been observed (Harman, 1981). Restricting the release of free radicals by means of a diet is supposed to have a favourable effect on cardiovascular diseases and diseases of the central nervous system, in particular atherosclerosis and hypertension (Harman, 1981). During the process of brain aging, lipofuscin would play an important role; anti-oxidants would reduce the release of lipofuscin (Harman, 1981). Swaab (1991) indicates that lipofuscin is no longer considered as a contributor to the aging process. Neurons of the hypothalamus which do not contain lipofuscin still show considerable degeneration during aging (Swaab, 1991).

Aging coincides with changes in the central nervous system, making the central nervous system more vulnerable for neurodegenerative diseases. These neurodegenerative diseases cause inactivity which, together with aging, contributes to changes in the various sensory systems, for example the motor system. The changes in the sensory systems will further increase inactivity and accelerate the aging process. This vicious circle (figure 1) could be interrupted at the level of the sensory systems, by enhancing for example the level of physical activity.

Indeed, there is now evidence that the level of e.g., physical activity is associated with the level of cognitive function. More specifically, the higher the level of physical activity the lower is the risk of Alzheimer's disease (Rovio et al., 2005). Physical activity but also other types of neuronal stimulation are encompassed in an enriched environment. The favourable effect of an enriched environment on the brain metabolism has been paraphrased as 'use it or lose it' (Swaab, 1991).

'Use it or lose it'

Brain aging is not only associated with loss of neurons (Swaab, 1991; Swaab et al., 1998). Instead, brain aging is characterized by atrophy which implies shrinkage of neurons. Shrunken cells still possess some metabolism and neurons with a reduced metabolism become vulnerable for neurodegenerative diseases such as Alzheimer's disease (Swaab, 1991).

Aging and Alzheimer's disease are not only characterized by degenerative processes but also by regeneration (Swaab, 1991; Swaab et al., 1998). It has been observed that loss of neurons in aging and even in Alzheimer's disease can be compensated by an increase in dendrites (Coleman & Flood, 1987). These findings show that plastic changes are still possible during aging and Alzheimer's disease (Swaab, 1991). Stimulation of neurons plays an important role in this process. The hypothesis that neuronal stimulation (e.g., enriched environment) might slow down the progression of neurodegenerative diseases and initiate regenerative processes in aging and Alzheimer's disease, has been paraphrased as 'use it or lose it' (Swaab, 1991). Swaab (1991) indicates four possible ways by which neuronal stimulation could take place: exposure to enriched environment and manipulation of trophic factors, hormones, and neurotransmitters.

The 'use it or lose it' hypothesis has been criticized as well as supported. One criticism is that excitatory neurotransmitters like glutamate play an important role in learning and memory, but that glutamate hyperactivity is neurotoxic and may lead to a reduction in dendrites and to cell death (Greenamyre, 1991; Mattson, 1991; McEwen, 1991; Sapolsky, 1991; Sofroniew, 1991). It is, therefore, important to keep neuronal activation within its normal physiological limits (Swaab, 1991). Advocates of the 'use it or lose it' concept emphasize that the quality of the interaction with the environment is essential for neural plasticity (Black, Isaacs, & Greenough, 1991). Exposure to an enriched environment should take place in life as early as possible. Such an early experience would create a kind of 'neuronal reserve' which could face up to the degeneration which accompanies aging. Of note is that sprouting only contributes to neuroplasticity and hence to a therapeutic effect when it occurs in an early stage of Alzheimer's disease (Geddes & Cotman, 1991). Sprouting during the course of Alzheimer's disease may produce plaques. Another support for the 'use it or lose it' concept is that the primary sensory areas are relatively preserved during aging and Alzheimer's disease, whereas these areas are active from the very beginning of life.

Taken together, the age-related reduced metabolism in the brain, strengthened by a decline of various types of sensory stimulation, makes the brain vulnerable for the occurrence of neurodegenerative diseases like Alzheimer's disease. Despite the severity of the neuropathology in Alzheimer's disease, regenerative processes may still take place, for example by stimulating the brain by sensory stimuli of various modalities. Importantly, stimulating the brain must take place within certain limits.

1.2.4 Epidemiology of Vascular dementia

Next to Alzheimer's disease, vascular dementia is the second most prevalent subtype of dementia (Román et al., 2002; Román, 2004; Román & Kalaria, 2006). In Japan, 50% of the patients with dementia have vascular dementia (Román, 2004). In people above 85 years of age, vascular dementia might even be more common than Alzheimer's disease (Jellinger, 2002). Vascular dementia occurs most frequently in men, in contrast to Alzheimer's disease as mentioned earlier (Román & Kalaria, 2006).

Risk factors for vascular dementia include 1) hypo- and hypertension, 2) cardiovascular disease, 3) diabetes, 4) smoking, 5) age, 6) lower level of education, 7) lacunar strokes and 8) white matter lesions (Román et al., 2002). These risk factors indicate that in some instances, vascular dementia could be prevented. In other words, early identification of these risk factors, preferably in a preclinical stage, is extremely important because in that case preventive treatment strategies can be administered (Bowler, 2002).

1.2.5 Epidemiology of frontotemporal dementia

The little information that is available about the prevalence of frontotemporal dementia indicates is that the prevalence varies from 3.6 per 100.000 people (age range: 45 – 64 years of age) to 15 cases per 100.000 people (age range: 50 – 59 years of age) (Neary, Snowden, & Mann, 2005). In general, the prevalence of frontotemporal dementia is much lower than the prevalence of Alzheimer's disease (Neary et al., 2005).

Frontotemporal dementia includes three clinical syndromes, each syndrome with its own neuropathology: the 'frontal variant' of frontotemporal dementia, the 'temporal variant' of frontotemporal dementia, also called 'semantic dementia' (Seeley et al., 2005), and progressive aphasia (Neary et al., 2005). The course of the disease is much faster for the frontal variant of frontotemporal dementia than for Alzheimer's disease and mortality is significantly increased when patients with the frontal variant of frontotemporal dementia also suffer from amyotrophic lateral sclerosis (Roberson et al., 2005).

1.3 Neuropathology in Aging and Dementia

First, the basal forebrain, related areas and neurotransmitter systems will be briefly discussed. The reason is that the basal forebrain cholinergic complex consists of a group of neurons that not only play an important role in a more global functional circuit, the ascending reticular activating system (ARAS), but also shows degeneration in a variety of neurodegenerative disorders such as Alzheimer's disease, Parkinson's disease, Down's syndrome, Jakob-Creutzfeldt disease, Korsakoff's syndrome and Pick's disease (McKinney & Jacksonville, 2005). The involvement of the basal forebrain cholinergic neurons in neurodegenerative diseases illustrates its central role in brain functioning.

Subsequently, neuropathology such as atrophy, reduced metabolism, neuritic plaques, neurofibrillary tangles, neuronal loss, neurotransmitter deficits and reduced vascularisation will be discussed with respect to a few brain areas and related neurotransmitter systems that play an important role in the clinical manifestation of aging, MCI, Alzheimer's disease, vascular dementia, and frontotemporal dementia.

1.3.1 The basal forebrain, related brain areas and neurotransmitter systems

Basal forebrain and the cholinergic neurotransmitter system
The cortical cholinergic system originates from the basal forebrain. The septum, one of the basal forebrain areas, is a major cholinergic source for the hippocampus whereas the rest of the brain, including the amygdala, receives a cholinergic innervation from another basal forebrain nucleus, the nucleus basalis of Meynert (NBM) (Mesulam, 2004) (see figure 2). The cholinergic innervation of the thalamus originates from the pedunculopontine tegmental nucleus (Mesulam, 2004).

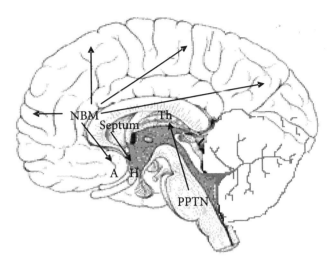

Figure 2. Cholinergic pathways from the septum to the hippocampus (H), from the nucleus basalis of Meynert (NBM) to the amygdala and other cortical areas, and from the pedunculopontine tegmental nucleus (PPTN) to the thalamus (Th).

Other neurotransmitter systems

The basal forebrain also receives serotonergic, noradrenergic, and cholinergic input from lower level brain stem areas such as the dorsal raphe nucleus, the locus coeruleus, and the pedunculopontine tegmental nucleus, respectively (Bobillier et al., 2001). These three brain stem areas, origins of the serotonergic, noradrenergic, and cholinergic neurotransmitter systems (Engelborghs & DeDeyn, 1997), are part of the ARAS (Kayama & Koyama, 1998). Interestingly, the locus coeruleus and the dorsal raphe nucleus project to the basal forebrain (Bobillier et al., 1976), and together with the pedunculopontine tegmental nucleus to the prefrontal cortex, the hippocampus, the amygdala, and the hypothalamus (Bobillier et al., 1976; Florin-Lechner, Druhan, Aston-Jones, & Valentino, 1996; Kocsis & Vertes, 1992; Legoratti Sanchez, Guevara-Guzman, & Solano-Flores, 1989; Marcyniuk, Mann, & Yates, 1986; Robbins & Everitt, 1995; Vertes, 1991).

In sum, the basal forebrain/cholinergic system plays a central role in the cooperation between brainstem areas and brain areas such as the prefrontal cortex, the striatum, and the hippocampus which are involved in higher cognitive processes.

1.3.2 Aging

The neuropathology of aging, Mild Cognitive Impairment (MCI), Alzheimer's disease, vascular dementia, and frontotemporal dementia will be briefly discussed with respect to atrophy, reduced metabolism, neuritic plaques, neurofibrillary tangles, neuronal loss, neurotransmitter deficits, and reduced vascularisation.

Atrophy and reduced metabolism

The normal cognitive aging process of the brain is characterized by a selective instead of a more global degeneration process (Raz, Torres, & Spencer, 1993). Atrophy occurs primarily in the frontal and temporal lobe and in the amygdala-hippocampal region of older persons without dementia (Coffey et al., 1992). In comparison with Alzheimer's disease, other cortical areas would show much less neuropathology during aging (Arriagada, Marzloff, & Hyman , 1992). Also others observed an age-related decline in the posterior frontal lobe (DeCarli et al., 1994) which is related to the quantity of white matter in the frontal lobe compared to the temporal lobe. There is more white matter in the frontoparietal cortex (45%) than in the temporal cortex (33%) and aging particularly influences white matter (see 'vascularisation'). Another example of 'selective' aging is that the prefrontal, polymodal association areas are more sensitive for the aging process than the primary somatosensory and visual cortex (Brody, 1992; Raz et al., 1993). Of note is that the prefrontal cortex needs most time for development and is the most vulnerable for aging (Lalonde & Badescu, 1995).

Keller (2005) describes pathological features in the aging brain that may have a negative effect on cell metabolism and thus enhance atrophy. These features are argyrophilic grains, lipofuscin, neuromelanin, and corpora amylacea. Argyrophilic grains are intracellular protein aggregates, presented as intraneuronal lesions. Argyrophilic grains occur primarily in the neuropil and have been observed in cortical areas such as the entorhinal cortex, in the amygdala complex but also in the hypothalamus (nucleus tuberalis lateralis). Argyrophilic grains damage neurons in a way similar to neurofibrillary tangles, for example it hinders the normal functioning of tau (argyrophilic grains are mainly composed of tau). Lipofuscin is composed of protein and lipid and occurs in, among others, the hippocampus. Neuromelanin contains lipofuscin but also produces lipofuscin, occurs primarily in the substantia nigra and locus coeruleus, and increases throughout life. It is not clear whether neuromelanin has a damaging or a beneficial effect on a cell. Corpora amylacea are cytoplasmatic, glycoproteina-cous inclusions, can be observed as astrocytes, and are found in, among others, the basal ganglia, the hippocampus, and the spinal cord. The presence of corpora amylacea may be beneficial, but may also damage cell metabolism. The number of corpora amylacea shows a remarkable increase in Alzheimer's disease (Keller, 2005).

Neuritic plaques, neurofibrillary tangles, and neuronal loss

In general, older persons show diffuse plaques whereas neuritic plaques and neurofibrillary tangles are characteristic for patients with Alzheimer's disease. However, already in normal aging Alzheimer-related neuropathology occurs (Fernando & Ince, 2004). This group may be viewed as 'presymptomatic Alzheimer patients'. There is some limited neuronal loss in the hippocampus but not widespread over the whole brain (Keller, 2005). An age-related loss of neurons has also been observed in the cerebellum (Andersen, Gundersen, & Pakkenberg, 2003). Neuronal loss has also been found in brain stem areas such as the locus coeruleus (Brody, 1992; Coleman & Flood, 1987; Manaye, McIntire, Mann, & German, 1995).

Neurotransmitter deficits, vascularisation

The degeneration of the prefrontal cortex during aging can also be attributed to an age-related decline in the dopaminergic, noradrenergic, and cholinergic neurotransmitter systems (McGeer et al., 1990), the latter through degenerative changes in the basal forebrain (Zhang, 2004). At the brain stem level, neuronal loss has been observed in the locus coeruleus/noradrenergic system (Brody, 1992; Coleman & Flood, 1987; Manaye et al., 1995). The consequence is that the level of noradrenalin in higher level areas connected to the locus coeruleus also reduces: a decline in noradrenalin was observed in the NBM, the basal ganglia, the hypothalamus, the fronto temporal cortex, the hippocampus, and the visual cortex (Pascual et al., 1991). A reduction in noradrenalin has not been observed in the amygdala indicating again that aging is not a generalized, global degenerative process. Also in the dorsal raphe nucleus/serotonergic system, neuronal loss has been observed in aging. This finding emerges from a study with old rats (28 months) (Lolova & Davidoff, 1991). These authors highlight the relationship between degeneration of the dorsal raphe nucleus and serotonergic neurons in the neocortex, the hippocampus and some areas of the basal ganglia. Little is known about the effect of aging on the pedunculopontine tegmental nucleus.

Results from animal experimental studies with very old rats show that the deficit in the NBM/cholinergic system may negatively influence the vascularisation of the brain during aging (Uchida, Suzuki, Kagitani, & Hotta, 2000). This phenomenon has been called 'neuronal vasodilatation'. Particularly a decrease in the nicotinic-receptor activity, and not in the muscarinic-receptor activity, may reduce the cerebral blood flow in the frontal and parietal lobe (Uchida et al., 2000; Sato, Sato, & Uchida, 2002) (figure 3). Focal electrical stimulation of the NBM increased the cortical cerebral blood flow in old rats but to a much lesser extent in very old rats (Sato et al., 2002). In line with these findings is the observation that in people not older than 60 years of age the neurovascular cerebral autoregulation appears to be unaffected (Rosengarten, Aldinger, Spiler, & Kaps, 2003).

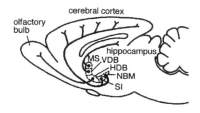

Figure 3 Reprinted with permission from Sato, A., Sato, Y., & Uchida, S. (2002). Regulation of cerebral cortical blood flow by the basal forebrain cholinergic fibers and aging. Autonomic Neuroscience: Basic and Clinical, 96, 13-19. Elsevier Science, Amsterdam.

The decline in the cortical cerebral blood flow by a cholinergic neural dysregulation may be responsible for the cognitive impairment in old age and Alzheimer's disease (Sato et al., 2002).

Cerebral vascular disease occurs in older persons with and without dementia in such a way that it hardly discriminates between both groups (Fernando & Ince, 2004). In that study, small vessel disease occurred in 64% older persons without dementia and in 75% older persons with dementia (Fernando & Ince, 2004). Of note is that cardiovascular risk factors such as hypertension particularly influence the white matter by decreasing vascularisation (Román et al., 2002).

1.3.3 Mild Cognitive Impairment (MCI)

Atrophy and reduced metabolism
A recent MRI study showed that the volume of the hippocampus highly discriminated between MCI patients and those without cognitive impairment (Wolf et al., 2004). More specifically, MCI patients show a clear reduction in the hippocampal volume. The global brain atrophy is not more pronounced in MCI, compared to older persons without dementia (Wolf et al., 2004). Of note is that the significant atrophy of the hippocampus is characteristic for amnestic MCI patients and not for multi-domain MCI (Becker et al., 2006). This is an important finding suggesting that multi-domain MCI should not be considered as a more advanced stage of amnestic MCI (Becker et al., 2006). The former group has extensive cortical atrophy (Becker et al., 2006). Furthermore, atrophy of the posterior region of the corpus callosum has been observed in MCI (Wang et al., 2005). Finally, MCI patients might also show a hypoperfusion of the inferior right parietal lobe (Johnson et al., 2005).

Neuritic plaques, neurofibrillary tangles, and neuronal loss
Results of recent studies indicate significantly elevated neuritic plaques in the frontal, parietal, and temporal neocortical region and the amygdala and neurofibrillary

tangles in the parietal neocortical region and in ventromedial temporal lobe structures such as the amygdala, entorhinal cortex, CA1 and subiculum (Markesbery et al., 2006). A high density of neurofibrillary tangles has been confirmed in temporal regions such as the entorhinal cortex, the gyrus fusiformis, the inferotemporal gyrus, and the temporal lobe (Guillozet, Weintraub, Mash, & Mesulam, 2003).

Neurotransmitter deficits
Alzheimer-related neuropathology, such as neurofibrillary tangles, affects the basal forebrain/cholinergic system in MCI (Mesulam, Shaw, Mash, & Weintraub, 2004). It has been hypothesized that the cholinergic deficit would particularly damage hippocampal function (Grön, Brandenburg, Wunderlich, & Riepe, 2006). Indeed, the cholinesterase inhibitor galanthamine improved exclusively episodic memory, a function in which particularly the hippocampus is involved (Grön et al., 2006).

Vascularisation
In a recent study, MCI patients who developed Alzheimer's disease showed a reduced blood flow in bilateral parahippocampal gyri, precunei, posterior cingulate cortex, bilateral parietal association areas, and the right middle temporal gyrus (Hirao et al., 2005).

1.3.4 Alzheimer's disease

Atrophy and reduced metabolism

Atrophy
The cortical frontal, temporal, parietal, and occipital lobes are characterized by atrophy (Regeur, Jensen, Pakkenberg, Evans, & Pakkeberg, 1994; Swaab, Hofman, Lucassen, Salehi, & Uylings, 1994; Swaab et al., 1998). As can be seen from figure 4 and figure 5, atrophy means shrinkage of neurons and not primarily cell death. An MRI study showed that atrophy of the hippocampus (medial temporal lobe) highly differentiates between normal aging and Alzheimer's disease (Jack, Petersen, O'Brien, & Tangalos, 1992). MRI is able to measure structural changes in the hippocampus even before clinical symptoms are noticeable (Fox et al., 1996). In that study, neither the person himself nor the family were aware of any cognitive impairment although a decline in memory could be assessed (Fox et al., 1996).

Subcortical areas that are severely affected in Alzheimer's disease are for example the basal forebrain among which the septum and the NBM (Swaab, 2003, 2004). The septum projects to, among others, the hippocampus, and the NBM to the cerebral cortex (Cummings & Back, 1998; Wenk, 2003) (see 'neurotransmitters'). Areas of the basal forebrain also project to the hypothalamus and to the hypothalamic suprachiasmatic nucleus (SCN) (Höhmann, Antuono, & Coyle, 1988), the 'biological clock' of the brain. In addition, brain areas such as the locus coeruleus, dorsal raphe nucleus and the pedunculopontine tegmental nucleus (PPTN) are severely affected in Alzheimer's disease (Braak & Braak, 1991). Consequently, the ARAS is affected in Alzheimer's disease (O'Mahoney, Rowan, Feely, Walsh, & Coakley, 1994).

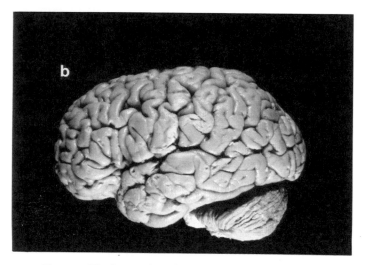

Figure 4. The brain of an older person without dementia.
With permission of the Netherlands Institute of Brain Research.

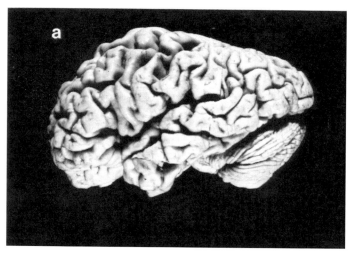

Figure 5. The brain of an Alzheimer patient.
With permission of the Netherlands Institute of Brain Research.

Reduced metabolism

There is ample evidence for reduced metabolism in Alzheimer's disease, reflected in a deterioration of mitochondrial enzyme activity (Sullivan & Brown, 2005). Mitochondria play a pivotal role in the production of adenosine triphosphate (ATP), a phosphate necessary for energy-demanding actions. Reduced metabolism has been observed in the frontal cortex, middle frontal gyrus, and the temporoparietal cortex. Importantly, reduced metabolism may precede neuropathology such as cerebral atrophy and neurological function (figure 6). It is noteworthy that the primary somatosensory areas show a lower reduction in glucose metabolism than the primary auditory, visual and motor areas (Arriagada et al., 1992; Blesa et al., 1996).

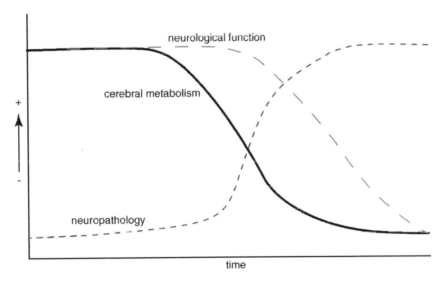

Figure 6. A theoretical model that shows that a decrease in cerebral metabolism precedes Alzheimer-related neuropathology and the loss of neurological function (Sullivan & Brown, 2005). Reprinted with permission from Sullivan, P.G., & Brown, M.R. (2005). Mitochondrial aging and dysfunction in Alzheimer's disease. Progress in Neuro-Psychopharmacology & Biological Psychiatry, 29, 407-410. Pergamon-Elsevier Science, Oxford.

Neuritic plaques, neurofibrillary tangles, and neuronal loss

Alzheimer's disease is characterized by extracellular neuritic amyloid plaques and intraneuronal neurofibrillary tangles. These neuropathological features occur preferably in the cerebral cortex, in particular in the temporal and parietal lobes (Braak & Braak, 1991). Neuritic plaques and neurofibrillary tangles are found in the entorhinal cortex in the initial stages of Alzheimer's disease. During its course these neuropathological features occur in the hippocampus and all other cortical areas except in the primary sensori-motor areas. In the final stage neuritic plaques are also found in subcortical areas such as the striatum, the thalamus, and the hypothalamus (Braak & Braak, 1991). It is noteworthy that not all brains of Alzheimer patients contain neuritic plaques and neurofibrillary tangles (Fernando & Ince, 2004). The amyloid cascade hypothesis implies that amyloid plaques become neuritic plaques by an inflammatory process These neuritic plaques constitute neurofibrillary tangles which are neurotoxic and lead to cell death (Gotz, Schild, Hoerndli, & Pennanen, 2004). A major criticism on this hypothesis is that in the entorhinal cortex the quantity of amyloid does not parallel the number of neurofibrillary tangles, the number of lost neurons and the stage of the disease (Swaab et al., 1998). Swaab and co-workers (1998) emphasize that amyloid should only be considered as one of the risk factors for Alzheimer's disease. In boxers with an Alzheimer-type dementia, amyloid plaques and neurofibrillary tangles have been observed in the hippocampus, in the absence of neuritic plaques. In other words, neuritic plaques and neurofibrillary tangles occur in the brain independent from each other. It is doubtful whether amyloid plaques are always transformed into neuritic plaques (Swaab et al., 1998).

A few examples of brain areas which are known for neuronal loss in Alzheimer's disease are the frontal cortex, the middle temporal gyrus, the entorhinal cortex, the parahippocampal cortex, the hippocampus and the locus coeruleus (Coleman & Flood, 1987; Swaab et al., 1998; Sullivan & Brown, 2005).

Neurotransmitter deficits

In Alzheimer's disease quite a number of neurotransmitters are affected such as acetylcholine, noradrenalin, serotonin, dopamine, somatostatin, and glutamate (Wenk, 2003). One of the neurotransmitter systems most severely affected in Alzheimer's disease is the cholinergic system (Wenk, 2003); this issue will be addressed first. Next, the relationship between the cholinergic and the serotonergic and between the noradrenergic and the serotonergic system will be discussed.

Cholinergic neurotransmitter system

There is ample evidence that the cholinergic system is affected in an advanced stage of Alzheimer's disease but probably also in an early stage in view of the cholinergic loss in the temporal lobe of aged people without dementia (Mesulam, 2004). It might be harder to detect a cholinergic deficit in an early stage of Alzheimer's disease since the control group with whom they will be compared, may also show a cholinergic deficit. One way to determine a cholinergic deficit is by counting the cholinergic neurons. The finding that a cholinergic deficit plays a crucial role in Alzheimer's disease is supported by the beneficial effects of cholinesterase inhibitors.

Loss of cholinergic neurons has been observed in the cerebral cortex; the entorhinal cortex, hippocampus, amygdala are the most severely affected while the primary sensory-motor areas are the least affected (Mesulam, 2004; Wenk, 2003). Cholinergic deficits have also been observed in the medial prefrontal (attention) and inferior parietal cortex (graphomotor ability) (Mesulam, 2004). A decline in memory may not only be due to a loss of cholinergic neurons considering the presence of plaques and tangles in the aforementioned areas. On the other hand, a cholinergic deficit could initiate the production of amyloid and the formation of neurofibrillary tangles, although a causal relationship between a deficit in the cholinergic system and the formation of amyloid plaques and tangles is weak (Mesulam, 2004).

With respect to pathways, loss of cholinergic neurons has been observed in the pathway projecting from the septum, one of the areas of the basal forebrain (Garcia-Alloza et al., 2005), to the hippocampus and in the pathway coming from the NBM projecting to the cerebral cortex (Wenk, 2003) (see figure 7). At this point, we refer to the 'functional circuits' described in the next chapters in which the prefrontal cortex, the entorhinal cortex/hippocampus and the parietal lobes play a pivotal role.

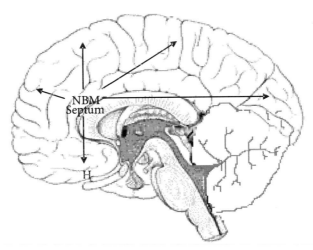

Figure 7. Cholinergic projection from the basal forebrain to the cerebral cortex. More specifically, cholinergic projection from the septum to the hippocampus (H) and from the nucleus basalis of Meynert (NBM) to the cerebral cortex.

Cooperation between the cholinergic and serotonergic neurotransmitter systems
There is a close cooperation between different neurotransmitter systems. For example, the cholinergic and serotonergic neurotransmitter systems are working

close together (Garcia-Alloza et al., 2005). They hypothesized that an imbalance between the cholinergic and serotonergic neurotransmitter system in the cerebral cortex would cause a cognitive decline and behavioural disturbances such as psychosis, overactivity, aggressive behaviour and depression (Garcia-Alloza et al., 2005). In particular, they argue that by a cholinergic deficit neuronal systems become more vulnerable for other neurotransmitter deficiencies such as the serotonergic system. A deficit in both systems would then be responsible for the cognitive and behavioural deficits. The results show a marked depletion of both the cholinergic system and the serotonergic system in the frontal and temporal lobe. Interestingly, however, the clinical outcome differs according to which neurotransmitter system is affected (see figure 8). Low cholinergic activity was associated with aggressive behaviour and cognitive impairment; a serotonergic deficit in the frontal cortex was associated with overactivity, in the temporal cortex with psychosis (Garcia-Alloza et al., 2005). In other words, not only the type of neurotransmitter but also the location of the neurotransmitter deficit in the brain determines its contribution to cognitive and/or behavioural disturbances (see figure 8).

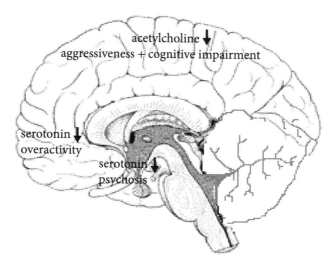

Figure 8. A deficit in the cholinergic system causes aggressive behaviour and cognitive impairment; a serotonergic deficit in the frontal lobe causes overactivity, in the temporal lobe a psychosis. ↓ = a deficit.

Cooperation between the noradrenergic and serotonergic neurotransmitter systems
An interaction between the noradrenergic and serotonergic system has been examined with respect to axonal regeneration in adult rats (Liu, Ishida, Shinoda, & Nakamura, 2003). Liu and co-workers (2003) observed that noradrenergic axons re-

generated well when the serotonergic axons were denervated, implying that in the normal situation serotonergic axons have an inhibitory effect on the regenerative process of noradrenergic neurons. Interestingly, however, the regeneration of serotonergic axons was hampered in the absence of noradrenergic neurons, indicating that noradrenergic axons are a prerequisite for the regeneration of serotonergic axons (Liu et al., 2003).

A reciprocal connection between the dorsal raphe nucleus/serotonergic system and the locus coeruleus/noradrenergic system has also been observed in a recent animal experimental study (Kim, Lee, Lee, & Waterhouse, 2004). The findings of that study show that the serotonergic projection from the dorsal raphe nucleus is stronger to the locus coeruleus than vice versa.

Vascularisation

Results from a recent study show that the majority of the Alzheimer patients suffered from vascular pathology in the brain (Fernando & Ince, 2004). Vascular problems in Alzheimer's disease may be expressed as cerebral amyloid angiopathy (CAA) which could be viewed as a combination of pathology typical for Alzheimer's disease (amyloid) and vascular pathology (angiopathy). CAA concerns the deposition of protein in the blood vessel walls of the brain (Castellani, Smith, Perry, & Friedland, 2004), among which the amyloid β-precursor protein. The involvement of the amyloid β precursor protein in CAA underscores a relationship between vascular problems and Alzheimer's disease (Castellani et al., 2004). Of note is that CAA causes ischemia and haemorrhage (Castellani et al., 2004). Cerebral ischemia initiates the degeneration and death of neurons (Koistinaho & Koistinaho, 2005). A consequence might be that the cognitive decline in Alzheimer's patients with CAA is much more severe than without CAA (Castellani et al., 2004). Of note is that a considerable number of Alzheimer patients show evidence of cerebral infarcts and that the presence of cerebrovascular disease aggravates the course of Alzheimer's disease. One of the underlying mechanisms might be that brain ischemia may enhance inflammatory processes by inducing pro-inflammatory mediators (Koistinaho & Koistinaho, 2005); their release is enhanced on the basis of among others oxygen deprivation. The reverse is also possible: the presence of Alzheimer neuropathology may increase the risk for cerebrovascular disease (Koistinaho & Koistinaho, 2005). Patients with Alzheimer's disease may later develop a stroke. Alzheimer's disease may also develop without CAA.

Vascular pathology might also cause white matter lesions. Compared to subcortical white matter lesions, periventricular white matter lesions prevail the most (Fernando & Ince, 2004) in both older persons with and without dementia.

1.3.5 Vascular dementia

Atrophy

The most prevalent subtype of vascular dementia is subcortical ischemic vascular dementia (Román et al., 2002). The pathological sequence of events underlying subcortical ischemic vascular dementia as follows: hypertension causes a disease of the small vessels (arteriolosclerosis) which subsequently causes either an occlusion or hypoperfusion. An occlusion leads to a complete infarction, also called a lacunar infarction ('Lacunar state'); hypoperfusion creates an incomplete infarction which damages the white matter, a disease entity called 'Binswanger's disease' (see figure 9).

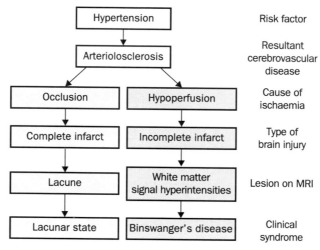

Figure 9. A pathological sequence of events underlying Lacunar state and Binswanger's disease: due to hypertension, arteriolosclerosis causes either an occlusion or hypoperfusion, resulting in a complete or incomplete infarct, respectively. Reprinted with permission from Román, G.C., Erkin-juntti, T., Wallin, A., Pantoni, L., & Chui, H.C. (2002). Subcortical ischaemic vascular dementia. Lancet Neurology, 1(7), 426-436. Lancet Ltd, London.

Importantly, to develop vascular dementia, a clinical stroke needs not to be part of the medical history of the patient (Knopman et al., 2003). The severity of the dementia is more associated with atrophy of the hippocampus and the cerebrum, than with white matter lesions (Román et al., 2002). In other words, atrophy of the hippocampus is not only characteristic for Alzheimer's disease (Bowler, 2002). White matter lesions severely affect frontosubcortical, in particular frontostriatal circuits (Pugh & Lipsitz, 2002) (see also Chapter 2).

The white matter lesions can be divided into periventricular and intracortical/subcortical white matter lesions. These types of white matter lesions have a different effect on cognitive functioning: periventricular white matter lesions have a more profound negative effect on cognition (de Groot et al., 2002).

Neuritic plaques, neurofibrillary tangles, and neuronal loss

In a recent clinicopathological study it was observed that if the brains of demented patients showed vascular lesions, the frontal and temporal lobes of those brains contained less amyloid plaques, neuritic plaques, and neurofibrillary tangles (Zekry et al., 2002). Also others found in some rare cases neuritic Alzheimer-type neuropathology in the brains of patients with vascular dementia (Jellinger, 2002). One of the consequences of the above described infarctions is neuronal loss, for example in the hippocampus (Jellinger, 2002).

Neurotransmitter deficits

A cholinergic deficit, expressed by a reduction in choline acetyltransferase activity (a marker for cholinergic activity), has been demonstrated in patients with vascular dementia, independent of Alzheimer neuropathology (Román, 2004). The cholinergic deficit is not so prominent as in Alzheimer's disease (Román & Kalaria, 2006). The question arises why a cholinergic deficit occurs in patients with vascular dementia. Areas of the cholinergic basal forebrain, for example the septum, are penetrated by small arteries and are therefore most vulnerable for hypertension (Román, 2004). Patients with vascular dementia also show infarctions of the NBM (Román & Kalaria, 2006). In addition, lesions in the white matter and basal ganglia which also have a cholinergic innervation, may disrupt the frontosubcortical cholinergic circuits. Moreover, the cholinergic connection between the nucleus NBM and for example the amygdala (figure 2) is vulnerable in patients with vascular dementia (Román, 2004). Of course, other neurotransmitter systems may be involved, dependent on the location of the lesion(s).

Vascularisation and reduced metabolism

The cholinergic system, originating from among others the NBM, activates a vasodilatory system, resulting in an increase in cerebral blood flow (Román, 2004). This relationship appears to be reciprocal: the cerebral blood flow also influences the functioning of the cerebral cholinergic neurons (Román & Kalaria, 2006). In other words, stimulating one system may thus have a beneficial effect on the other. A decline in cerebral blood flow is reflected in a decrease in for example glucose metabolism (Román & Kalaria, 2006).

1.3.6 Frontotemporal dementia

Frontotemporal dementia is linked to chromosome 17 and is characterized by dementia and parkinsonism (van Swieten et al., 1999). Patients with frontotemporal dementia are classified as patients with Pick's disease (Kersaitis, Halliday, & Kril, 2004). The neuropathology is quite specific for frontotemporal dementia (for a review, see Munoz et al., 2003) and does not show an overlap with Alzheimer's disease nor with vascular dementia. Nevertheless, for sake of comparison with Alzheimer's disease and vascular dementia, atrophy, reduced cerebral blood flow, reduced metabolism, neuronal loss, and neurotransmitter deficits will be briefly discussed in two variants of frontotemporal dementia: the 'frontal variant' and the 'temporal variant'

1.3.7 The 'frontal variant' of frontotemporal dementia

Atrophy and reduced metabolism
In contrast to Alzheimer's disease and vascular dementia, the most severe atrophy was observed in the frontal, lateral anterior temporal, and parietal regions (Varma et al., 2002a). More specifically, in the early stage, atrophy has been found in the frontal cortex and hippocampus (Kersaitis et al., 2004). In some cases, atrophy of the temporal lobe is even more pronounced than that of the frontal lobe (Neary et al., 2005). White matter lesions have been seen in frontotemporal dementia but to a lesser extent than in vascular dementia (Varma et al., 2002b). Reduced metabolism has been observed in the right medial prefrontal cortex, orbitoprefrontal cortex and anterior cingulate cortex (Varrone et al., 2002).

Neuronal loss
In an early stage, neuronal loss is particularly found in the frontal cortex. During the course of the disease also the temporal lobe, particularly the hippocampus, shows neuronal loss (Kersaitis et al., 2004).

Neurotransmitter deficits
Due to a deficit in the serotonergic neurotransmitter system, glucose metabolism is declining in the frontal lobe (Franchesi et al., 2005). In line with this finding is the observation of hypoperfusion in the left superior frontal cortex (Osawa et al., 2004). The involvement of the serotonergic system in this disorder has been confirmed by others (Yang & Schmitt, 2001). In that study, the locus coeruleus/noradrenergic system appeared to be spared in frontotemporal dementia. This latter finding is not supported by others (Munoz et al., 2003). Furthermore, an impair-

ment in the nigrostriatal dopaminergic system has been observed (Rinne et al., 2002).

1.3.8 The 'temporal variant' of frontotemporal dementia

Atrophy
Atrophy has been observed in the ventromedial prefrontal cortex (Seeley et al., 2005). Moreover, atrophy of the hippocampus has been found (van de Pol et al., 2005), although not confirmed in each study (Hodges, 2001).

Neuronal loss
Neuronal loss has been found in the anterior and inferior temporal lobe, particularly in the left hemisphere (Davies et al., 2005), in the parahippocampal gyrus and in the fusiform gyrus (Davies, Graham, Xuereb, Williams, & Hodges, 2004; Chan et al., 2001a).

1.4 Summary

Alzheimer's disease and vascular dementia, in particular subcortical ischemic vascular dementia, are two of the most common causes of dementia. Table 1 shows the major neuropathological characteristics of aging, Mild Cognitive Impairment, Alzheimer's disease, vascular dementia, and frontotemporal dementia, i.e., the frontal and temporal variant.

A major difference between aging, Mild Cognitive Impairment and Alzheimer's disease is that neuritic plaques and neurofibrillary tangles are typical for Mild Cognitive Impairment and Alzheimer's disease. Atrophy, reduced metabolism, neurotransmitter deficits, neuronal loss, a decline in vascularisation, and white matter lesions do occur in aging but to a much lesser extent than in Alzheimer's disease. Although neuritic plaques and neurofibrillary tangles have been observed in vascular dementia, the main difference is the cerebrovascular disease in vascular dementia, as reflected in Lacunar State and Binswanger's disease. Despite the fact that frontotemporal dementia has its own specific neuropathology, both the frontal and temporal variant of frontotemporal dementia show an overlap with the other subtypes of dementia and aging with respect to atrophy, reduced metabolism, neuronal loss, and white matter lesions. A striking similarity between all the presented subtypes of dementia is the involvement of the (pre)frontal cortex and the hippocampus (see table 1).

Neuropathological characteristics of aging and the various subtypes of dementia

	Atrophy	Reduced metabolism	Neurotransmitter deficits	Plaques/ NPs/NFTs	Neuronal loss	Decline in vascularisation/ cerebral blood flow	White matter lesions
Aging	Association areas Frontal/temporal Amygdala/ Hippocampus	Entorhinal cortex Amygdala Hypothalamus Substantia nigra Locus coeruleus	Acetylcholine Dopamine Noradrenaline Serotonine	Plaques	Hippocampus (limited) Cerebellum LC	present	periventricular
MCI							
AD	Frontal, temporal, parietal, occipital Hippocampus Basal forebrain Hypothalamus LC, DRN, PPTN	Frontal lobe Temporo-parietal lobe Primary auditory, visual, motor areas	Acetylcholine Noradrenaline Serotonine Dopamine Somatostatin Glutamate	NPs, NFTs in cortex (temporal, parietal) Entorhinal cortex Hippocampus Striatum Thalamus Hypothalamus	Frontal cortex Middle temporal gyrus Entorhinal cortex Parahippocampal cortex Hippocampus LC	CAA	periventricular
VaD	Hippocampus Cerebrum		Acetylcholine Other neurotransmitters, dependent on location of lesion	Frontal + temporal lobes, less than in AD	e.g. hippocampus NBM Basal ganglia	Lacunar State Binswanger's disease	Particularly Binswanger's disease frontostriatal systems
FTD 'frontal' variant	Frontal lobe Anterior temp. lobe Parietal lobe Hippocampus	Right medial PFC Orbitofrontal Anterior cingulate	Noradrenaline Dopamine ?		Frontal cortex Temporal cortex Hippocampus		Frontal lobe (less than in VaD)
FTD 'temporal' variant	Ventromedial PFC Hippocampus				Anterior/inferior Temporal lobe Parahippocampal gyrus Gyrus fusiformis		

Table 1. Neuropathological characteristics of aging and the various subtypes of dementia. NPs: neuritic plaques; NFTs: neurofibrillary tangles; MCI: Mild Cognitive Impairment; AD: Alzheimer's disease; VaD: vascular dementia; FTD: frontotemporal dementia; LC: locus coeruleus; DRN: dorsal raphe nucleus; PPTN: pedunculopontine tegmental nucleus; CAA: cerebral amyloid angiopathy; temp.: temporal; PFC: prefrontal cortex; NBM: nucleus basalis of Meynert.

1.5 Questions

1.   Mention six risk factors for Alzheimer's disease.
2.   Is there a relationship between level of education and the risk for Alzheimer's disease?
3.   What is meant by 'apoptosis'?
4.   Why does 'short weight' have a beneficial effect on the aging process?
5.   Could you describe the 'vicious circle of accelerated aging'?
6.   On which neuropathological feature of Alzheimer's disease is the 'use it or lose it' hypothesis based upon?
7.   Mention four possible ways by which neuronal stimulation might take place.
8.   Under which circumstances could glutamate weaken the 'use it or lose it' hypothesis?
9.   Is sprouting always a favourable outcome of neuronal stimulation?
10.   Mention eight risk factors for vascular dementia.
11.   Which three clinical syndromes are encompassed by frontotemporal dementia?
12.   Could you briefly describe the central role of the basal forebrain/cholinergic system in the functioning of the brain?
13.   Which neurotransmitter system is strongly associated with the basal forebrain?
14.   Which brain area provides one of the major cholinergic inputs of the hippocampus?
15.   Mention three brainstem areas and related neurotransmitter systems that project to the basal forebrain.
16.   In which brain regions shows white matter the highest prevalence?
17.   Is the normal cognitive aging process a more global or a more specific degeneration process?
18.   Does age have a differential effect on primary and polymodal association areas?
19.   Which lobes are particularly vulnerable for aging?
20.   Which brainstem area in humans shows a strong age effect?
21.   What is meant by 'neuronal vasodilatation'? Which neurotransmitter system is particularly involved in the reduction in cerebral blood flow in people older than 60 years of age?
22.   Atrophy of a specific medial temporal lobe structure differentiates best between normal aging and Alzheimer's disease; which area?
23.   Could you explain the interaction between reduced metabolism, atrophy, and neurological function in Alzheimer's disease?
24.   What is the main criticism on the amyloid cascade hypothesis?
25.   Which neurotransmitter systems are involved in Alzheimer's disease?
26.   Which brain areas of Alzheimer patients are the least affected by a loss of cholinergic neurons?
27.   Which two 'functional circuits' are characterized by a loss of cholinergic neurons?
28.   What is the effect of a cholinergic deficit on behaviour in Alzheimer's disease?
29.   The effect of a cholinergic deficit on behaviour appears to depend on the location in the brain. Please explain.
30.   What is meant by CAA? What is the relationship/interaction between cerebrovascular disease and Alzheimer's disease?
31.   Please explain the difference in neuropathology between Lacunar state and Binswanger's disease.

32. Do neuritic plaques and neurofibrillary tangles occur in vascular dementia?
33. Describe the major neuropathological differences between the frontal and the temporal variant of frontotemporal dementia.

Chapter 2
Functional circuits in cognitive aging and Mild Cognitive Impairment

2.1 Introduction

We will all agree: if we are growing older, we would like to stay independent as long as possible. Cognitive functions that are involved in the maintenance of this independency are 'executive functions' (Pugh & Lipsitz, 2002). There is no consensus about the nature and the number of cognitive functions executive functions are composed of. Heyder and colleagues (2004) distinguish the following elements of these hierarchical spoken highest cognitive functions (Duke & Kaszniak, 2000), i. e., the performance of more than one task simultaneously (divided attention), set-shifting (disengaging attention and focusing attention on a new stimulus) and inhibition (the suppression of irrelevant stimuli in order to focus attention to relevant stimuli). According to Lezak (1995) executive functions include the following cognitive capacities: 1) taking initiatives, goal setting and motivation ('volition'), 2) planning, 3) purposive action and self-regulation, and 4) efficient performance. Irrespective of the concept of executive functions that one wants to use, it is clear that the prefrontal cortex (PFC) is one of the brain areas that plays a major role in executive functions (Fassbender et al., 2004).

Executive functions coordinate and control other cognitive functions such as episodic memory (Erickson & Barnes, 2003), a function that is traditionally strongly related to the functioning of the hippocampus (Eldridge, Engel, Zeineh, Bookheimer, & Knowlton, 2005). A strong functional relationship between the PFC and the hippocampus (Ericson & Barnes, 2003) is reflected in the important role that attention and inhibition play in episodic memory (Aron, Robbins, & Poldrack 2004; Rossi et al., 2004; Carbeza, Anderson, Locantore, & McIntosh, 2002). After all, one has to be able to focus attention on the information one wants to remember and one has to be able to suppress (inhibit) irrelevant information.

The PFC and the hippocampus are involved in executive functions and episodic memory. These areas are part of a larger 'functional circuit' which is affected by age. In this chapter several functional circuits and a limited number of related brain areas will be described. Subsequently, discussing the influence of age on these circuits and related brain areas, makes it possible to explain age effects on certain aspects of executive functions and episodic memory. In the same way, the relationship between functional circuits, executive functions, episodic memory, and Mild Cognitive Impairment (MCI) will be presented.

Taken together, this chapter focuses on two important and related cognitive functions, i.e., executive functions and episodic memory, for the following reasons:

1) executive functions and episodic memory play a major role in independent functioning in daily life activities (Cahn-Weiner, Boyle, & Malloy, 2002; Ward, 2003).

2) executive functions, episodic memory, and involved brain areas such as the PFC and hippocampus, respectively, are most vulnerable for aging (Braver & Barck, 2002; Uylings & de Brabander, 2002; Raz et al., 2005).

3) a description of particularly these two specific cognitive functions instead of a large number of cognitive functions facilitates the explanation of the clinical symptoms that are characteristic for aging and MCI (this chapter) but are also characteristic for the various subtypes of dementia such as Alzheimer's disease, vascular dementia, and frontotemproal dementia (next chapter).

2.1.1 *Several 'specific' functional circuits*

Functional circuits are the result of the activation of various brain areas (grey matter) which cooperate with each other by pathways (white matter) which connect the various brain areas

Grey matter. Within the scope of executive functions, the PFC – a cortical brain area – is working close together with areas situated in lower parts of the brain (subcortical) such as the striatum, one of the regions of the basal ganglia (figure 1). The resulting 'frontostriatal circuit' is innervated by among others the dopaminergic system which has its origin in another subcortical area, the substantia nigra (nigrostriatal system) (Nieoullon, 2002; Bäckman & Farde, 2001).

Moreover, with respect to executive functions, the PFC shows a profound cooperation with the anterior cingulate cortex (ACC) and the cerebellum (figure 1) (Diamond, 2000; Heyder, Suchan, & Daum, 2004); the latter is called the 'frontocerebellar circuit'.

The nigrostriatal system not only innervates the PFC but also the hippocampus (Nieoullon, 2002). At a functional level, exchange of information takes place between the hippocampus and PFC through the entorhinal cortex (figure 2), called the 'frontohippocampal circuit'. The cooperation between the PFC and hippocampus contributes to attention and working memory (Erickson & Barnes, 2003). There also exists a parahippocampal-hippocampal stream; the parahippocampal cortex is connected with the parietal cortex and the thalamus, two areas that are involved in visuospatial functions (Erickson & Barnes, 2003).

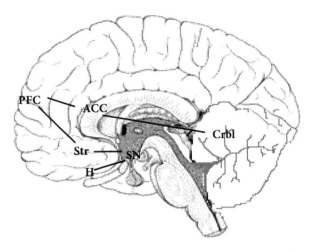

Figure 1. 'Functional circuits' that play an important role in executive functions and episodic memory include the frontostriatal system, the nigrostriatal system, and connections between the prefrontal cortex (PFC) and the anterior cingulate cortex (ACC) and the cerebellum (Crbl). Str: striatum; SN: substantia nigra (dopaminergic system); H: hippocampus.

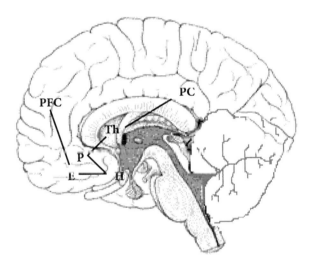

Figure. 2. Functional circuits that play a role in attention, working memory and visuospatial functions include connections between the hippocampus (H) and prefrontal cortex (PFC) through the entorhinal cortex (E), and between the parahippocampal cortex, hippocampus, thalamus (Th) and parietal cortex (PC).

White matter. White matter can be divided into two subtypes: white matter around the ventricles, called 'periventricular white matter', and white matter that connects cortical areas (intracortical) and cortico-subcortical areas that lie at a short distance from each other, called 'subcortical white matter' (de Groot et al., 2002). Periventricular white matter consists of long pathways that are situated along and around the ventricles while subcortical white matter consists of short U-shaped pathways (Filley, 1998) (figure 3).

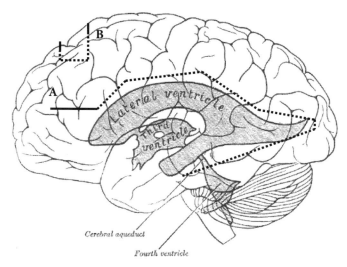

Figure 3. An example of (A) periventricular white matter: long pathways connecting areas that lie at a long distance from each other and (B) subcortical white matter which connects closely situated cortical areas with each other through short U-shaped loops. Closed lines: cortical; interrupted line: subcortical.

In sum, the striatum sends strong afferent projections to the PFC (frontostriatal circuit) and the hippocampus. The hippocampus itself has a strong functional relationship with the PFC (frontohippocampal circuit) and the parietal cortex. These areas are connected with each other by white matter, which can be divided into periventricular and subcortical white matter.

2.1.2 An 'aspecific' functional circuit

Not every functional circuit plays a specific role in cognitive functions such as executive functions. A well-known example of a system that contributes to the functioning of the central nervous system in a more global way is the ascending reticular activating system (ARAS) (Kayama & Koyama, 1998). By controlling the level of activity of the whole brain, the contribution of the ARAS is more aspecific (Robbins & Everitt, 1995). This level of activity is also called 'arousal'. Brain areas that play an essential role in the ARAS and thus in arousal are situated at a sub-cortical level of the central nervous system, more particular at the brain stem level (Kayama & Koyama, 1998). Brain stem areas that play a crucial role in the ARAS are the locus coeruleus (LC), the dorsal raphe nucleus (DRN), and the pedunculo-pontine tegmental nucleus (PPTN) (figure 4) (Kayama & Koyama, 1998). These three brain stem areas are the sources of ascending neurotransmitter systems, i.e., the noradrenergic, the serotonergic, and the cholinergic neurotransmitter system, respectively (Kayama & Koyama, 1998).

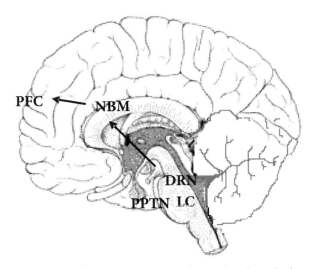

Figure 4. The Ascending Reticular Activating System (ARAS) with, at the lowest level, brain stem areas such as the locus coeruleus (LC), dorsal raphe nucleus (DRN) and the pedunculopontine tegmental nucleus (PPTN), through the nucleus basalis of Meynert (NBM), the ARAS reaches the prefrontal cortex (PFC). Reprinted with permission from Petrides, M., & Milner, B. (1982). Deficits on subject-ordered tasks after frontal and temporal-lobe lesions in man. Neuropsychologia, 20 (3), 249-262. Pergamon-Elsevier Science, Oxford.

It has been established that both the noradrenergic and the serotonergic system demonstrate the highest activity while being awake. Interestingly, however, the increased activity in each of these two systems has a different effect on higher level areas (Robbins & Everitt, 1995): the noradrenergic system activates, the serotonergic system inhibits (Kayama & Koyama, 1998). With respect to arousal, the DRN/ serotonergic system and the LC/noradrenergic system relate to each other in a very specific way (Quick & Sourkes, 1977): the DRN/serotonergic system has an inhibiting influence on the LC/noradrenergic system to prevent overarousal (Jacobs, Heym, & Trulson, 1981; Kayama & Koyama, 1998). In other words, interactions between the DRN/serotonergic and LC/noradrenergic system are necessary to keep the arousal level in balance.

The LC and DRN project to the basal forebrain (Bobillier et al., 1976), in particular to the nucleus basalis of Meynert (NBM), an area that is the origin of the cortical cholinergic system (Ezrin-Waters & Resch, 1986). Considering the projection of both neurotransmitter systems to the NBM, one can understand that the cooperation between the noradrenergic and serotonergic system during arousal may also be mediated through the cholinergic neurons of the NBM. In a study, the effects of the LC/noradrenergic system and the DRN/serotonergic system on the cholinergic basal forebrain neurons were examined in vivo in rats (Cape & Jones, 1998). The results show that through the NBM/cholinergic system, noradrenalin increases EEG activity whereas EEG activity is reduced by serotonin. EEG activity is representative for the level of cortical activity (arousal) (Cape & Jones, 1998). By this mediating role and by the widespread and diffuse projections to the neocortex and the hippocampus (Dunnett & Fibiger, 1993), the NBM/cholinergic system is considered a further continuation of the ARAS (Mesulam, 1995; Richardson & De-Long, 1988). Indeed, the results of animal experimental studies show that the NBM/cholinergic neurons play an important, more aspecific, role in attention and arousal, instead of a role in specific memory processes (Voytko, 1996).

Finally, the LC and DRN, together with the PPTN, project to the PFC (Florin-Lechner, Druhan, Aston-Jones, & Valentino, 1996; Vertes, 1991; Robbins & Everitt, 1995). The PFC is considered one of the cortical target areas of the ARAS (see figure 4) (Robbins & Everitt, 1995). Of note is that the PFC is the only structure with a descending influence on brain areas such as the LC, DRN and PPTN (Robbins & Everitt, 1995). Through this feedback system, particularly the right PFC plays a crucial role in the suppression of irrelevant stimuli (Casey et al., 1997; Jonides, Smith, Marshuetz, Koeppe, & Reuter-Lorenz, 1998; Strik, Fallgatter, Brandeis, & Pascual-Marqui, 1998). Suppression (inhibition) of irrelevant stimuli creates the possibility to focus attention to relevant information which enhances executive functions such as cognitive flexibility (Baddeley & Wilson, 1988).

Taken together, the ARAS is an aspecific functional circuit which has its origin in a number of brain stem areas that show a strong projection to the basal forebrain, in particular the NBM, with the PFC as one of the cortical target areas. Serotonergic, noradrenergic, and cholinergic neurotransmitter systems are involved in the ARAS. The ARAS plays an important role in the maintenance of the level of activity of the brain, also called arousal.

2.2 Normal aging

2.2.1 *Functional circuits*

Brain areas belonging to specific functional circuits
Results of a number of studies show that those areas that play an important role in executive functions such as the PFC, the striatum and the cerebellum, are vulnerable for aging (Salat et al., 2004; Raz, Rodrique, Head, Kennedy, & Acker, 2004). A longitudinal study of 5 years showed that most atrophy was observed in structures such as the striatum and the cerebellum with similar degeneration in the PFC and prefrontal white matter, the connecting pathways between the various brain areas (Raz et al., 2003, 2005).

An interesting suggestion which is supported by literature is that tertiary, associative cortical brain areas such as the PFC and the cerebellum are areas that finish their development the latest (Diamond, 2000; Fuster, 2002) and are the most vulnerable for aging (Raz et., 2005). However, this 'last in, first out' phenomenon is weakened by the finding that thinning (atrophy) of the primary visual and motor cortex was not less than the atrophy of the PFC (Salat et al., 2004). Furthermore, studies show that not the whole PFC is affected by aging. In one study using Magnetic Resonance Imaging (MRI) a significant reduced volume of the PFC was observed in older people in comparison with younger people, except for the orbitofrontal cortex which was preserved in the older population (Salat, Kaye, & Janowsky, 2001). In contrast, another fMRI study showed that during the performance of a memory task (remembering a word that had just been presented) one specific area within the PFC (Brodmann's area 9) was extra vulnerable for aging (Johnson, Mitchell, Raye, & Greene, 2004). Aging also affects the ACC (Barnden, Behin-Ain, Kwiatek, Casse, & Yelland, 2005). Among the different brain areas in the medial temporal lobe, the age effect on the hippocampus is much stronger than on the entorhinal cortex (Raz et al., 2004). This is an important finding since, as mentioned earlier, the hippocampus communicates with the PFC through the entorhinal cortex (Erickson & Barnes, 2003).

One of the factors which is involved in the observed atrophy during aging is that the hippocampus is less sensitive for growth factors (neurotrophins). Growth factors such as neurotrophin3 (NT-3) play a major role in the development of the hippocampus (Smith, 1996). The activity of the nigrostriatal dopaminergic system shows an age effect; as has been stated before, the nigrostriatal dopaminergic neurons innervate the PFC and the hippocampus (Reeves, Bench, & Howard, 2002).

Lesions in the white matter during aging occur especially in the frontal areas (Head et al., 2004). This phenomenon is related to the quantity of white matter in these brain areas. White matter prevails more in the frontoparietal cortex (45%)

than in the temporal cortex (33%) (DeCarli et al., 1994). Interestingly, the onset of Alzheimer's disease does not coincide with an increase in white matter lesions in the anterior regions but much more in the posterior regions (Head et al., 2004). This finding implies that the neurophysiologic mechanisms underlying aging are not the same as those underlying Alzheimer's disease (Head et al., 2004). Based upon cardiovascular risk factors such as hypertension, age, and diabetes mellitus, white matter lesions during aging are often the result of problems in the small blood vessels (Buckner, 2004; Pugh & Lipsitz, 2002). It should be realized, however, that small to moderate white matter lesions may occur in older persons who do not show signs of a neurological disease (Desmond, 2004).

The nature of white matter lesions – periventricular or subcortical – is important with respect to cognitive functioning. Subjective cognitive complaints, assessed by means of a questionnaire, show the strongest relationship with disorders of the periventricular white matter, compared to disorders of the subcortical white matter (de Groot et al., 2001). The importance of this finding is that subjective cognitive complaints could be an important predictor for the development of dementia in a later stage (de Groot et al., 2001). Moreover, more white matter lesions were observed in those people who indicated to experience a progressive decline in cognitive functioning. The same research group performed a longitudinal study over a period of 10 years (de Groot et al., 2002). In this longitudinal study the relationship was measured between the level of periventricular and subcortical white matter lesions and the rate of cognitive decline. The age of the participants was between 60 and 90 years of age. Level of cognitive functioning was measured by means of the Mini-Mental State Examination (MMSE) (Folstein, Folstein, & McHugh, 1975). The results show that only the level of periventricular white matter lesions was associated with the rate of cognitive decline. A possible explanation for this large age effect on the periventricular white matter is that the vascular architecture (vascularisation) of the periventricular white matter is more sensitive to age-related diseases such as, for example, atherosclerosis (Pantoni & Garcia, 1997). Probably influenced by hypertension, a high correlation has been observed between a decline in prefrontal white matter and atrophy of the hippocampus (Raz et al., 2005). Also a recent MRI-study is interesting in which old-old people (mean age: 85.5 years!) participated (Piguet et al., 2003). In that study, the relationship between white matter lesions (periventricular and subcortical) and cognitive functioning was examined. An extensive neuropsychological test battery was administered and white matter lesions were assessed in frontal, temporal, parietal, and occipital areas. The results show that specifically periventricular white matter lesions occur in older persons. A striking finding is that no relation was observed between periventricular white matter lesions and the performance on the majority of the cognitive tasks. There was no association between executive functions and 'frontal' white matter lesions, neither periventricular nor subcortical. For three of the neuropsychological tests, a 'threshold-effect' was observed for white matter lesions which implies that white matter lesions should be present in a certain quantity before correlations with cognitive performance can be observed. An important conclusion is that white matter lesions in the old-old people has no influence on cognitive functioning in a way as observed in young people (Piguet et al., 2003). An explanation might be that at this age the brain had time to prepare itself for these changes and, consequently, had time to develop compensatory strategies.

Pugh & Lipsitz (2002) notice that the various fronto-subcortical circuits which are involved in either cognition or motor activity, are situated so close together that it is quite logical that cognitive and motor disturbances occur together. A decline in motor activity expresses itself in extrapyramidal signs such as bradykinesia (slowing of movements) and disturbances in gait, fine motor activity and balance (Pugh & Lipsitz, 2002). White matter lesions could also be the cause of emotional disorders like depression, mania and disinhibition (Pugh & Lipsitz, 2002).

Taken together, specific functional circuits which play a role in executive functions and episodic memory are vulnerable for aging. Brain areas that play a prominent role in these functional circuits are the PFC and the hippocampus. With respect to the pathways connecting brain areas, periventricular and subcortical white matter lesions differ in their effect on cognition. The former disturbs cognition the most. The effect of white matter lesions on cognitive functioning in the old-old is restricted.

The aspecific functional circuit

The white matter lesions discussed before also affect the functioning of the ARAS. Moreover, at the brain stem level, neuronal loss has been observed in the LC (Brody, 1992; Coleman & Flood, 1987). The consequence is that the level of noradrenalin in higher level areas which are connected to the LC also declines during aging. Indeed, an age-related decline in noradrenalin was observed in among others the NBM, the basal ganglia, the fronto-temporal cortex and the hippocampus (Pascual et al., 1991). A decline in noradrenalin was not observed in the amygdala, supporting the view that aging has an influence on specific brain areas and does not concern a more global, generalized process (Pascual et al., 1991).

Neuronal loss has also been observed in the DRN. These results parallel those of a study with old rats (28 months of age) (Lolova & Davidoff, 1991). These authors emphasize the relationship between degeneration of the DRN and degeneration of serotonergic neurons in the neocortex, hippocampus, and nuclei of the basal ganglia. Little is known about the effect of aging on the PPTN/cholinergic system (see figure 5). Results from another animal experimental study with rats show that the age effect observed in this nucleus does not influence cognition (Gill & Gallagher, 1998).

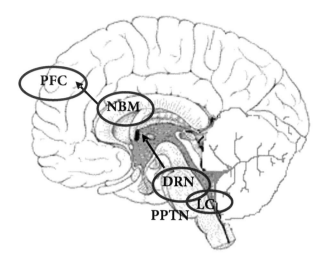

Figure 5. Areas of the Ascending Reticular Activating System (ARAS) that are affected by age (circled): LC: locus coeruleus, DRN: dorsal raphe nucleus, NBM: nucleus basalis of Meynert, PFC: prefrontal cortex. Little is known about the effect of age on the PPTN (pedunculopontine tegmental nucleus).

2.2.2 Cognitive decline in aging

Executive functions

As has been discussed before, executive functions are the product of a cooperation between various brain areas and their connections and should not be exclusively associated with the functioning of the (pre)frontal lobe (Heyder et al., 2004). The question arises whether the clinical manifestation of aging depends on where in the functional circuit, e.g., the frontostriatal circuit, the decline is the most pronounced. A decline in PFC functioning expresses itself in an impairment in divided attention, set-shifting, and inhibition. The precise contribution of the ACC to executive functions remains obscure (Heyder et al., 2004). A decline in the functioning of the striatum has an effect on executive functions, speed of information-processing, and episodic memory (Bäckman & Farde, 2001). For people with a decline in the functioning of the striatum, dividing attention across tasks, each composed of another sensory modality, is very difficult (Heyder et al., 2004). The effect of age on the fronto-striatal system was also reflected in a reduction in inhibition (Sweeney, Rosano, Berman, & Luna, 2001). Concerning the frontocerebellar circuit: a decline in the functioning of this circuit provokes problems particularly in the speed of dividing attention between information of different sensory nature. Divided attention is also impaired during the performance of a motor task together with the detection of sensory signals like sounds (Heyder et al., 2004); for example, when an older person crosses the street. There is no evidence for a role of the cerebellum in inhibition.

So far, the influence of the dysfunctioning of one of the brain areas (grey matter) belonging to specific functional circuits on executive functions has been discussed. However, white matter lesions affect the connections between the various brain areas. As highlighted before, the nature of the white matter lesions (periventricular or subcortical) determines the clinical outcome. The results of several studies indicate that white matter lesions, in particular periventricular white matter lesions, impair executive functions (Desmond, 2004; Gunning-Dixon & Raz, 2000). White matter lesions are particularly responsible for hypometabolism in the PFC (Reed et al., 2004). The reduced metabolism in the PFC correlated not only with impaired executive functions but also with an impairment in memory and more global cognitive capacities. Reduced metabolism in the temporal lobe was associated with an impairment in memory and global cognitive functioning but not with an impairment in executive functions (Reed et al., 2004).

Importantly, a decrease in executive functions, among which attention, may depend on the extent to which white matter lesions occur (Desmond, 2004). According to Desmond, white matter lesions must reach a certain threshold beyond which they impair cognition.

Taken together, executive functions are vulnerable for aging, as a result of deterioration of both grey and white matter. The PFC and subcortical areas such as the striatum contribute differently to executive functions; for example, an impairment in inhibition is less pronounced with lesions in the PFC than with lesions in the striatum. Among all the areas that are involved in functional circuits, the PFC is the most sensitive for white matter lesions.

Episodic memory

Compared to executive functions, episodic memory shows the largest impairment as a result of the aging process (Burke & MacKay, 1997). In particular verbal episodic memory is sensitive to aging, possibly because a word yields less additional information that may contribute to encoding than, for example, a face (Bäckman, Jones, Berker, Laukka, & Small, 2004). It has been found that the performance shows a progressively larger age effect when the task is becoming more and more difficult, for example by presenting new, unknown material, by increasing the quantity of information to be remembered or by presenting the stimuli at a much faster rate (Burke & MacKay, 1997). One explanation for the impairment in episodic memory is that older people have problems in making new relationships between for example words to be remembered and the context in which the words were presented (Burke & MacKay, 1997). If these relationships are necessary to process recent and new information, then the performance in episodic memory of the older person declines whereas the performance on an episodic memory task remains at the same level when such new relationships are not required (Burke & MacKay, 1997). Another finding with respect to episodic memory is that, compared to men, women are much better in memorizing a list of groceries and names (West, Crook, & Barron, 1992). The most obvious explanation is that women, more than men, are better practiced in remembering list of groceries and have a richer social life, training them in remembering a lot of names (West et al., 1992). In the same study, years of education, marital status, employment status, and depression had no significant influence on memory performance when age was controlled for (West et al., 1992).

Recognition memory – a type of episodic memory – can be divided into two variants: a more explicit, contextual recognition memory and recognition memory based on the familiarity with the former presented item (more implicit). In one study, the effect of age on these two subtypes of recognition memory was examined (Parkin & Walter, 1992). Context-related recognition has also been paraphrased as 'source memory' and means that one is able to recognize an item because one exactly knows where and when the item was learned (the context) (Parkin & Walter, 1992). Context is not involved in recognition based on familiarity with the item; one simply knows which item is correct. Recognition based on familiarity with the item has also been paraphrased as 'knowing' (Parkin & Walter, 1992). The results show that young people, appeal much more to the context in recognizing the correct items while older people show more 'knowing' responses (Parkin & Walter, 1992). Of note is that the impairment in source memory in older people is associated with the dysfunction of the frontal lobe (Paulesu, Frith, & Frackowiak, 1993). An important conclusion is that in view of the maintenance of 'recognition in general' in elderly people, implicit recognition memory may compensate for the loss of explicit recognition memory (Paulesu et al., 1993).

It is known that the hippocampus plays a crucial role in learning new information and in retrieving information from memory (Kennedy & Shapiro, 2004; Shiflett, Tomaszycki, Rankin, & de Voogd, 2004). More specifically, it was observed in one study that the volume of the hippocampus and learning of both visuospatial and non-visuospatial tasks showed an age effect (Driscoll et al., 2003). It is noteworthy that in older persons a smaller volume of the temporal lobe, in which the hippocampus is situated, is not always associated with a decreased performance on memory tasks. Older persons who perform beyond average on memory tasks rather show a smaller volume of the temporal lobe (van Petten et al., 2004). An explanation for this finding is that this smaller volume is a reflection of a most favorable development of the brain early in life, during which period ineffective synapses are removed (van Petten et al., 2004). The age effect on the hippocampus is also reflected in an impairment in the visuospatial memory (next to learning, which was tested by memorizing the location of exhibited objects in a museum (Erickson & Barnes, 2003). The main consequence of age-related atrophy of the hippocampus is not an impairment in the direct recall of just learned material but a disturbance in delayed recall; the memory performance declines when there is a time interval between learning and retrieval of the information from memory (Erickson & Barnes, 2003).

The results of a recent study show that white matter lesions have no effect on episodic memory of older persons without dementia (Sachdev, Wen, Christensen, & Form, 2005). White matter lesions do have a negative effect on tasks that appeal to motor capacities such as the Purdue Pegboard and grip strength. Moreover, a relationship between lesions in white matter, in particular subcortical white matter, and a decrease in physical condition was observed (Sachdev et al., 2005).

In sum, episodic memory is vulnerable for aging, especially when episodic memory is involved in remembering new and a lot of information, presented within limited time. Aging also has a negative influence on episodic recognition memory if recognition strongly depends on the context in which the information is presented. Primary the hippocampus but also the PFC are involved in episodic memory. It is interesting that a smaller volume of the hippocampus is characteristic for older persons who perform at a very high level.

Rate of information processing
Considering the role of the ARAS in arousal, the ARAS contributes more globally to the functioning of the central nervous system (Robbins & Everitt, 1995). Damage to this system (see figure 5) may cause a decrease in the level of activity of the brain, resulting in slower and less flexible cognitive functioning. These two clinical symptoms are characteristic for normal aging (Burke & MacKay, 1997; Woodruff-Pak, 1997) and can be explained by two mechanisms (Salthouse, 1996). In the first place, some cognitive processes take place so slowly that after a certain time mistakes occur. In the second place, information from different channels enters the brain so slowly that the primary information has already disappeared at the moment the most recent information is processed. In other words, simultaneous processing of information is reduced in aging (Salthouse, 1996).

Preservation of cognitive functions in aging
Compared to executive functions, episodic memory, and rate of information processing, other cognitive functions such as language, and abstract reasoning are less vulnerable for aging (Small, Stern, Tang, & Mayeux, 1999). In addition, age appears to have little effect on procedural memory (Churchill, Stanis, Press, Kushelev, & Greenough, 2003). Similarly, an age effect has not been observed for driving a car,

writing and household activities (Erickson & Barnes, 2003). Results of a longitudinal study show that older persons are able to learn new complex motor tasks (with hands and fingers) and reproduce these new skills two years later without further training (Smith et al., 2005). Also short-term memory is relatively unaffected by age (Erickson & Barnes, 2003).

2.2.3 Mild Cognitive Impairment

Functional circuits

Brain regions belonging to specific functional circuits
One could argue that the vulnerability of the functional circuits in aging will increase in Mild Cognitive Impairment (MCI). However, as far as we know, a direct relationship between fronto-subcortical circuits and MCI has not been examined. A next question will then be which (sub)parts of these circuits (grey and white matter) are more affected in MCI than in normal aging. One area that meets these latter criteria is the hippocampus (Scheff, Price, Schmitt, & Mufson, 2005). Next to the hippocampus, more pronounced degeneration was also observed in the PFC and ACC of MCI patients compared to older persons without dementia (Johnson et al., 2004). Atrophy of the ACC is characteristic for those patients who later develop Alzheimer's disease (Chetelat & Baron, 2003). Of note is that a high prevalence of periventricular white matter lesions occurs in those MCI patients who do not progress into Alzheimer's disease but, instead, show a stable clinical picture (Maruyama et al., 2004).

The aspecific functional circuit
As far as the authors know, the relationship between brain stem areas involved in the ARAS and MCI has not been studied.

Executive functions
The assumption that, except for episodic memory, other cognitive functions such as executive functions, language, and praxis are completely preserved in MCI (Collie & Maruff, 2000) is somewhat surprising considering that already in normal aging functional circuits that are related to e.g. executive functions are impaired. A degeneration of the hippocampus, a neuropathological hallmark of MCI, interrupts the functional relationship between the hippocampus, the PFC and the parietal cortex (see figure 2). Indeed, the results of a recent study emphasize that an impairment in more than one cognitive function is characteristic for MCI (Bäckmann et al., 2004). Next to episodic memory, also the performance of tasks appealing to executive functions and perceptual speed highly contributes to a differentia-

tion between MCI and elderly people without dementia (Bäckman et al., 2004) (table 1).

Neuropsychological functions	Normal aging	Mild Cognitive Impairment
Episodic memory	+	++
Executive functions	+	++
Perceptual speed	+	++

Table 1. Cognitive functions that make a clear distinction between normal aging and Mild Cognitive Impairment (MCI). +:mildly affected; ++: more severely affected.

Episodic memory

In view of the influence of aging on episodic memory, it is not illogical that an impairment in this type of memory (memory for a story, learning a list of words) is also characteristic for people with MCI (Collie & Maruff, 2000). In the 'transitional stage' from normal aging to Alzheimer's disease (a number of MCI patients develop Alzheimer's disease; Jack et al., 1999), a strong correlation has been observed between an impairment in episodic memory and damage to the medial temporal lobe, in particular the hippocampus (Collie & Maruff, 2000). Chen and co-workers (2000) found that delayed recall of wordlists learned before (verbal episodic memory) made the best distinction between older people without cognitive impairment and those in a preclinical stage of Alzheimer's disease, i.e., MCI. Also the performance on Trailmaking B, a task appealing to executive functions, distinguishes very well between both groups. In other words, both episodic memory and executive functions will be affected already in a preclinical stage of Alzheimer's disease (Chen et al., 2000).

2.3 Summary

2.3.1 Specific functional circuits

By describing the various functional circuits (specific and aspecific) and the neuropathology of involved brain areas, insight is provided into the cognitive consequences of aging and MCI. Specific functional circuits which have been described include the frontostriatal circuit, the nigrostriatal circuit, a circuit consisting of connections between the PFC, ACC and cerebellum (frontocerebellar circuit), a circuit in which the hippocampus is connected to the PFC through the entorhinal cortex (frontohippocampal circuit), and a circuit in which the hippocampus, the thalamus and the parietal cortex are connected, through the parahippocampal cortex (see table 2).

Specific functional circuits	ARAS
Frontostriatal circuit	LC/noradrenergic system
Nigrostriatal circuit	DRN/serotonergic system
Frontocerebellar circuit	PPTN/cholinergic system
Frontohippocampal circuit	NBM/cholinergic system
Hippocampus – thalamus – parietal cortex	PFC

Table 2. Functional circuits (specific and aspecific) and related brain areas/neurotransmitter systems. PFC: Prefrontal cortex; ACC: anterior cingulated cortex; ARAS: Ascending Reticular Activating System; LC: locus coeruleus; DRN: dorsal raphe nucleus; PPTN: nucleus pedunculopontinus tegmentalis; NBM: nucleus basalis of Meynert.

2.3.2 Aspecific functional circuit

Brain areas that play a role in an aspecific functional system, the ARAS, are brain stem areas such as the LC/noradrenergic system, the DRN/serotonergic system, and the PPTN/cholinergic system. Higher level areas of the ARAS involve the basal forebrain, in particular the NBM/cholinergic system, and the PFC.

2.3.3 AGING

Age-related neuropathology of brain areas involved in the various functional circuits

Areas of the specific functional circuits that are affected in aging are the PFC, the ACC, the striatum, the hippocampus, and the cerebellum. In addition, age has an effect on periventricular white matter, in particular frontal white matter. Areas of the ARAS that are affected by age are the LC, DRN, and NBM (see table 3).

Brain areas belonging to the functional systems affected by aging	
Specific functional circuits	ARAS
PFC	LC
ACC	DRN
Striatum	NBM
Hippocampus	PFC
Cerebellum	

Table 3. Brain areas belonging to the functional systems that are affected by aging. PFC: prefrontal cortex; ACC: anterior cingulate cortex; ARAS: Ascending Reticular Activating System; LC: locus coeruleus; DRN: dorsal raphe nucleus; NBM: nucleus basalis of Meynert.

Cognitive decline in aging (see table 4)
Executive functions. Results of the clinical studies show that older persons show an impairment in executive functions, among which divided attention, set-shifting, inhibition, and in a (rapid) change of attention between different targets.

Episodic memory. Age also has a deteriorating effect on episodic memory, in particular when new material has to be learned, when it is a lot of information to be remembered, when the information is presentation at a much faster rate, and when the information has to be recalled after a delay of a certain amount of time. Moreover, 'source memory' (dependent on the context) and learning and memory of visuospatial tasks are vulnerable for aging.

Global cognitive functioning. Age slows down the rate and flexibility of information processing.

Cognitive decline in aging		
Executive functions	**Episodic memory**	**Global cognitive functioning**
Divided attention	New material	Speed of processing
(Rapid) change in attention	A lot of information Delayed recall	Flexibility
Set-shifting	Source memory	
Inhibition	Visuospatial learning and memory	

Table 4. Cognitive decline in aging.

Cognitive preservation in aging

Cognitive functions that are less affected by aging include language, visuospatial capacities, abstract reasoning, procedural memory, automatised activities of daily life, learning complex motor activities and short term memory.

2.3.4 Mild Cognitive Impairment (MCI)

MCI-related neuropathology of brain areas involved in the various functional circuits
Areas of the specific functional circuits that are affected in MCI include the PFC, ACC, and the hippocampus (see table 5). Also the periventricular white matter shows an age effect. Studies on the influence of MCI an areas of the ARAS have not been performed so far.

Brain areas belonging to the functional systems affected by MCI	
Specific functional circuits	**ARAS**
PFC	No information available
ACC	
Hippocampus	

Table 5. The influence of Mild Cognitive Impairment (MCI) on functional circuits. PFC: prefrontal cortex; ACC: anterior cingulate cortex; ARAS: Ascending Reticular Activating System.

Cognitive decline in MCI (see table 1)

Executive functions, episodic memory and speed of information processing (perceptual speed) deteriorate in MCI, more severely than in normal aging.

2.4 Questions

1. Mention four executive functions according to Lezak (1995).
2. Why is the relationship between the prefrontal cortex and the hippocampus so important for episodic memory?
3. What is the relationship between the substantia nigra and the frontostriatal circuit?
4. Which brain areas mediate an exchange of information between the hippocampus and the prefrontal cortex and between the hippocampus and the parietal cortex?
5. Mention two types of white matter and their location in the brain.
6. Where does the abbreviation 'ARAS' stand for? Why is its function more 'aspecific'?
7. Which brain stem areas and related neurotransmitters are part of the ARAS?
8. Which effect has the DRN/serotonergic system on the LC/noradrenergic system?
9. Which neurotransmitter system is closely related to the nucleus basalis of Meynert?
10. Mention one cortical target area of the ARAS.
11. What is meant by 'last in, first out' phenomenon in aging?
12. Which part of the prefrontal cortex is less and which part of the PFC is more vulnerable for aging compared to the other prefrontal areas?
13. Mention two age-related factors that negatively influence the functioning of the hippocampus.
14. Why does aging particularly influence the white matter in the frontal areas?
15. Do periventricular and subcortical white matter differ in their effect on cognition?
16. What is the relationship between white matter and subjective cognitive complaints?
17. What is the relationship between white matter and cognitive functioning in the old-old?
18. What is meant by a 'threshold effect' for white matter lesions?
19. Could you explain why disturbances in cognition and motor activity often occur together?
20. Could you provide some evidence that aging is not a global, generalized process?
21. Does it matter where in a specific functional circuit, e.g. the frontostriatal circuit, the deterioration is the most pronounced?
22. Does reduced metabolism in the PFC only affect executive functions?
23. Does reduced metabolism in the temporal lobe impair executive functions?
24. Which possible mechanism underlies the observed impairment in episodic memory in older people?
25. In which type of recognition memory is the frontal lobe particularly involved?
26. Is a smaller volume of the hippocampus always associated with as decreased performance on memory tasks?
27. What is the main cognitive consequence of age-related atrophy of the hippocampus?
28. Is slowness of information-processing in aging due to a decline in a specific functional circuit or in a aspecific functional circuit?
29. Mention a number of cognitive functions that are relatively preserved in aging.
30. Which cortical area (temporal lobe) shows early degeneration in Mild Cognitive Impairment (MCI)?
31. Which cognitive task made the best distinction between older people without cognitive impairment and those in a preclinical stage of Alzheimer's disease?
32. Which cognitive functions are most vulnerable in MCI?

Chapter 3
Functional circuits in dementia

3.1 Introduction

In this chapter I will continue with describing specific functional circuits, the aspecific functional circuit, executive functions and episodic memory, but now with respect to Alzheimer's disease, vascular dementia, and frontotemporal dementia, i.e., the frontal and temporal variant. First, however, a rather traditional classification of the various subtypes of dementia as either 'cortical' or 'subcortical' will be discussed. Such a classification is rather arbitrary, particularly within the scope of functional circuits which hallmark is the close cooperation between cortical and subcortical areas. Nevertheless, it helps understanding the clinical manifestation of the various subtypes of dementia as expressed in an impairment in episodic memory, in language/speech, in gross motor activity, and in behaviour and personality.

Since Alzheimer's disease is one of the most common causes of dementia, also other cognitive functions that will decline in Alzheimer's disease, next to executive functions and episodic memory, will be briefly summed up. At the end of the chapter, comparisons will be made between the frontal and temporal variant of frontotemporal dementia, and within the temporal variant of frontotemporal dementia between the neuropathology in the left and the right hemisphere. Additional comparisons will be made between frontotemporal dementia and Alzheimer's disease, and between Alzheimer's disease and vascular dementia. In comparing these disorders, the focus on executive functions and episodic memory will be abandoned and broadened with related cognitive functions and behaviour.

3.2 Functional circuits in 'cortical' versus 'subcortical' dementia

Traditionally, the various subtypes of dementia are classified either as 'subcortical' or 'cortical' dementia. For example, Alzheimer's disease has been labelled a cortical dementia because a main area that is affected already in a very early stage of the disease is the hippocampus (Ackl et al., 2005), which is a cortical area. In contrast, vascular dementia has been called subcortical dementia because its main neuropathology is characterized by a deficit in vascularization of subcortical brain areas such as the basal ganglia (Román, 2005). Therefore, the most prevalent subtype of vascular dementia is subcortical ischemic vascular dementia (SIVD) (Román, Erkinjuntti, Wallin, Pantoni, & Chui, 2002). Although a distinction between cortical and subcortical dementia may contribute to the understanding why certain clinical symptoms are characteristic for a specific subtype of dementia, such a classification is rather arbitrary for two reasons. In the first place, in Alzheimer's disease, a cortical subtype of dementia, also subcortical areas such as the locus coeruleus are affected, next to cortical areas (Zarow, Lyness, Mortimer, & Chui, 2003). In vascular dementia, a subcortical subtype of dementia, the frontal lobe is one of the most vulnerable brain regions (Román et al., 2002). In the second place, the hallmark of functional circuits (specific and aspecific) is that cortical and subcortical areas are working closely together, which implies that a lesion in one of the areas of the functional circuit will have its impact on the whole circuit.

However, from a neuropsychological (memory, language), motoric, and behavioural point of view it does matter if the primary lesion is situated in the cortical or subcortical area. Within this scope, it is interesting to briefly address the influence of cortical and subcortical dementia on episodic memory, language/speech, gross motor activity, and behaviour/personality.

Episodic memory. To test episodic memory, very frequently a list of unrelated words is read aloud to the patient who has to recall as many words as possible, directly after the presentation of the words but also after a delay. In case of a cortical lesion, the patient will not be able to encode and store the information in memory; encoding and storing information are true cortical functions. Consequently, if after a delay, the patient is asked to active recall as many words as possible from the list of words presented 10 minutes ago, the score will be low: the patient will not be able to retrieve the information from memory since it has not been stored in the cortex in the first place. Similarly, recognition of the words (the same list of words is read aloud again, but now mixed with words that have not been read aloud before), will probably not be much better. A prerequisite for a better recognition score than an active recall score is that the patient must have been able to store the information in the cortex but is not able to retrieve the information actively. With cortical lesions, the patient is neither able to actively reproduce the learned material nor to recognize it: 'amnesia'.

With subcortical lesions patients are much better able to store the words into memory because the cortex is relatively unaffected. The problem with subcortical lesions however is to retrieve that information from the memory store which implies that they, just like those with cortical lesions, show a low score in an active recall condition. However, the recognition score will be much higher than the active recall score in patients with subcortical lesions, compared to patients with cortical lesions (see table 1). After all, the words have been stored and can now be retrieved because they are presented once again. The memory deficit in these patients is best described as 'forgetfulness'.

Language/speech. Language is a higher-level cognitive function, requiring the co-operation of many cortical areas. Therefore language disturbances are characteristic for patients with a cortical lesion. However, in motor speech production, two distinct functional networks have been proposed (Riecker et al., 2005). A preparatory network including the mesiofrontal cortex, insula, and cerebellum is necessary to initiate movements. Another network includes brain areas such as the basal ganglia, thalamus, cerebellum and motor cortex; this network is necessary for the motor execution of speech, and activates the 'speech apparatus of the motor cortex' (Fabbro, Clarici, & Bava, 1996). (see figure 1). In other words, in speech production both cortical and subcortical areas are involved (see table 1).

	Cortical	Subcortical
Neuropsychological functions		
Failure to actively retrieve learned material	+	+
Amnesia	+	
Failure to recognize learned material	+	
Forgetfulness		+
Language disturbance	+	
Speech disturbance	+	+
Motor activity		
Deterioration of gross motor activity	+	++
Behaviour/personality		
Disinhibition (hyperactive)	+	
Depression/apathy		+

Table 1. Influence of cortical and subcortical lesions on neuropsychological functions, motor activity, behaviour/personality. + = present; ++ = more prominently present.

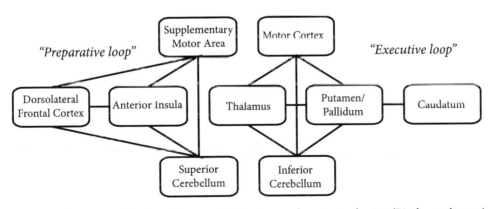

Figure 1. A 'preparatory loop' and 'an executive loop' in speech motor production (Riecker et al., 2005).

Gross motor activity. Basic motor activity is regulated by subcortical motor areas like the basal ganglia. It is noteworthy that also the striatum becomes affected in

Alzheimer's disease in a later stage (Braak & Braak, 1991) and may cause 'parkinsonian' symptoms such as rigidity (Funkenstein et al., 1993; Prehogan & Cohen, 2004; Wilson et al., 2000). In addition to subcortical areas, also the primary motor cortex is involved in Alzheimer's disease (Suva et al., 1999). 'Pseudoparkinsonian' symptoms may occur in Alzheimer's disease as well (for further reading, see chapter 6). Nevertheless, gross motor disturbances in Alzheimer's disease will not occur in an early stage but will become more prominent during its course.

Behavioural and personality symptoms. Cortical types of dementia are characterized by behavioural disturbances in physical behaviour like apathy, aberrant motor behaviour, and sleep disturbance (Mirakhur, Craig, Hart, McIlroy, & Passmore, 2004) and by behavioural/personality disturbances such as depression, anxiety, irritability/lability and agitation/aggression (Mirakhur et al., 2004). Aberrant motor behaviour, agitation, and irritability could also be viewed as signs of hyperactivity (Aalten et al., 2003) and could be due to a dysfunction of the prefrontal cortex (Franchesi et al., 2005). On the other hand, depression and apathy may be of subcortical origin. It is known that a deterioration in the noradrenergic, serotonergic, and dopaminergic neurotransmitter systems, which have their origin in the brain stem (Kayama & Koyama, 1998) and substantia nigra (dopaminergic system) (Chinta & Andersen, 2005), are involved in depression (Pacher & Kecskemeti, 2004). These brain areas are affected in Alzheimer's disease (see chapter 1). For a further explanation of the contrast between e.g., hyperactivity and apathy, please see the section 'Alzheimer's disease – executive functions'. Depression as a 'subcortical' disorder is indeed characterized by subcortical clinical symptoms such as forgetfulness instead of amnesia, recognition better than active retrieval from memory, improved memory performance by providing cues, stooped posture, and slowness in thinking and motor activity (Cummings & Benson, 1984; Caligiuri & Ellwanger, 2000) (see table 2).

Cognitive and motor disturbances in depression
Forgetfulness
Recognition of former learned material better than active retrieval from memory
Cues enhances memory
Slowness in thinking
Motor disturbances
Slowness in locomotion
Stooped posture

Table 2. Cognitive and motor disturbances characteristic for depression.

In sum, a distinction between cortical and subcortical dementias is arbitrary since the neuropathology of the most prevalent subtypes of dementia (Alzheimer's disease and vascular dementia) involves both cortical and subcortical areas. The clinical symptoms, which differ per subtype of dementia, depend on where in the functional circuits the neuropathology is the most severe. Against this background, the influence of Alzheimer's disease, vascular dementia, and frontotemporal dementia on the functional circuits and hence on executive functions and episodic memory, will be discussed.

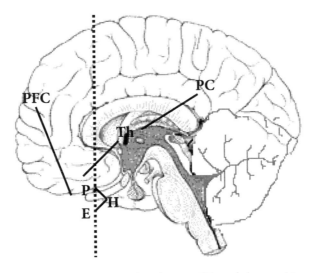

Figure 2. The hippocampus (H), the entorhinal cortex (E), and the parahippocampal cortex (P) are strongly affected in Alzheimer's disease, interrupting important specific functional circuits. PC: parietal cortex; PFC: prefrontal cortex; Th: thalamus.

3.3 Alzheimer's disease

Specific functional circuits
Brain areas that are affected in Alzheimer's disease play an important role in the former described functional circuits (chapter 2). Areas that show the most severe neuropathology, i.e., loss of neurons, already in a relatively early stage of Alzheimer's disease include the hippocampus (medial temporal lobe), and the entorhinal and parahippocampal cortex (Braak & Braak, 1991; Coleman & Flood, 1987; Uylings & Brabander, 2002). Consequently, the communication between the hippocampus and the prefrontal cortex mediated through the entorhinal cortex, and between the hippocampus and parietal cortex through the parahippocampal cortex, is severely disturbed (figure 2). A decrease in communication between neurons, and thus in cognitive functions, emerges not only from neuronal loss but also from a degeneration of dendrites and a decrease in the number of synapses (Uylings & Brabander, 2002).

The importance of an undisturbed communication between the hippocampus and the prefrontal cortex is illustrated by a recent PET-study (Grady, Furey, Pietrini, Horwitz, & Rapoport, 2001). This study shows that in memorizing faces for a short period, patients with Alzheimer's disease did not show a functional relationship between the right prefrontal cortex and the right hippocampus; such a relationship was present in older persons without dementia. Of note is that in patients with Alzheimer's disease cooperation exists between the various prefrontal areas during the performance of an episodic memory task (Grady et al., 2003).

Furthermore, a dysfunction of the nigrostriatal system has been observed in Alzheimer's disease (Pizzolato et al., 1996), interrupting the frontostriatal system and the connection between the nigrostriatal system and the hippocampus (figure 3). Indeed, the results of a recent study show that the dopaminergic receptors in the hippocampus are affected (Kemppainen et al., 2003).

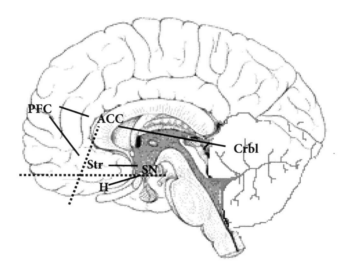

Figure 3. Disruption of nigrostriatal circuit interrupts the connection between the nigrostriatal circuit and the hippocampus and between the striatum and prefrontal cortex (frontostriatal system) H: hippocampus; SN: substantia nigra; Str: striatum; PFC: prefrontal cortex; ACC: anterior cingulate cortex; Crbl: cerebellum.

There is ample evidence that periventricular and subcortical white matter lesions occur in Alzheimer's disease (Scheltens & Kittner, 2000).

Taken together, the frontostriatal circuit, the nigrostriatal circuit, the fronto-hippo-campal circuit and the hippocampus – parietal circuit are damaged in Alzheimer's disease.

The aspecific functional circuit

Areas that play an essential role in the ARAS such as the locus coeruleus, dorsal raphe nucleus, pedunculopontine tegmental nucleus, the nucleus basalis of Meynert and the prefrontal cortex are all affected in Alzheimer's disease (see chapter 1).

Executive functions and episodic memory

Executive functions

As described in the section 'specific functional circuits', the prefrontal-hippocampal circuit is severely affected in Alzheimer's disease, with an emphasis on the hippocampal part of this circuit. In contrast, results from animal experimental and human studies suggest that the frontostriatal system may not be primarily damaged in Alzheimer's disease, although the striatum is involved during its course (Braak & Braak, 1991; Pizzolato et al., 1996). A recent study with transgenic Alzheimer mice shows that the preserved capacity for procedural learning even reflects an intact frontostriatal system, in the presence of hippocampal dysfunction (Middei, Geracitano, Caprioli, Mercuri, & Ammassari-Teule, 2004). The difference in impairment in these functional circuits suggests that an impairment in the performance of tasks that appeal primarily to executive functions will be present but less in comparison to the performance of tasks that depend heavily on episodic memory (see next section).

The performance of most cognitive tasks will, however, rely on an intact prefrontal-hippocampal circuit. In one study in which patients with Alzheimer's disease and patients with Huntington's disease participated, two types of word fluency tasks were administered: category fluency (animals and professions) and letter fluency (words starting with a specific letter) (Rosser & Hodges, 1994). Results of various studies show that in Alzheimer's disease particularly category fluency is affected (Diaz, Sailor, Cheung, & Kuslansky, 2004; Monsch et al., 1992; Rosser & Hodges, 1994; Marczinski & Kertesz, 2005). Category fluency is typically a task that appeals to both executive functions such as cognitive flexibility and productivity (prefrontal part of the circuit), and to an intact semantic and long-term episodic memory (hippocampal part of the circuit) (Pihlajamaki et al., 2000). In other words, for a good performance of category fluency, an intact prefrontal-hippocampal circuit is a prerequisite. Interestingly, it has been suggested that the performance of letter fluency depends on the functioning of another functional circuit, the frontostriatal system (Ho et al., 2002).

Alzheimer's disease is also characterized by a disturbance in planning, another executive function, which may express itself in an impairment in activities of daily life such as household activities. An example of a planning task is the Self-Ordered Pointing task (Petrides & Milner, 1982) (figure 4).

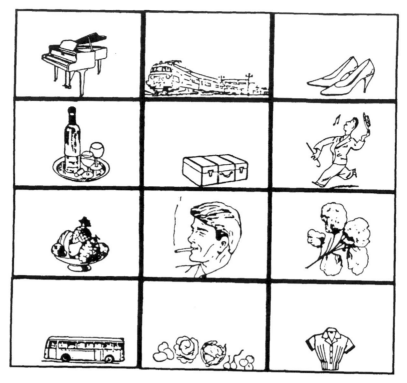

Figure 4. Self-Ordered Pointing task (Petrides & Milner, 1982).

Attention, working memory, abstract thinking and concept formation are executive functions that are also affected in Alzheimer's disease (Duke & Kaszniak, 2000). According to Lezak (1995), monitoring one's own behaviour plays a major role in the executive function 'efficient performance'. This requires a high level of disease insight and self-efficacy. There is ample evidence that Alzheimer patients underestimate their memory problems (Duke & Kaszniak, 2000). Lack of disease insight in Alzheimer's disease is due to a dysfunction of the frontal lobe.

Of note is that in Alzheimer's disease, disturbances in executive functions like taking initiatives, goal setting and motivation (also called 'volition') could be expressed as disturbances in behaviour and mood, for example apathy and depression (Duke & Kaszniak, 2000; Mirakhur et al., 2004). As mentioned earlier, also the reverse pattern is characteristic for Alzheimer's disease: hyperactivity, restlessness, and agitation, signs of disinhibition (Duke & Kaszniak, 2000; Mirakhur et al., 2004) (table 1). This diversity in clinical symptoms is also observed in vascular dementia and frontotemporal dementia. In contrast to the latter two disorders, in Alzheimer's disease these symptoms occur during the course of the disease, not before memory disturbances have been observed and are less prominent in comparison with frontal and fronto-subcortical disorders. It is argued that the contrast in clinical symptoms, i.e., apathy versus hyperactivity, is due to an imbalance between the dopaminergic (subcortical origin) and cholinergic (cortical origin) neurotransmitter systems. In case of a cholinergic deficit, the dopaminergic system transmission will be increased, causing hyperactivity (Gerber et al., 2001) whereas a loss of dopamine may produce apathy (Rémy, Mirrashed, Campbell, & Richter, 2005). Of note is that both neurotransmitter systems are involved in the frontostriatal system, in other words a misbalance in the frontostriatal system may be responsible for these clinical symptoms.

Episodic memory

Considering the vulnerability of the hippocampus and, consequently, episodic memory, for aging (chapter 2), it is not surprising that an impairment in episodic memory is one of the earliest and most prominent clinical symptoms in Alzheimer's disease (Almkwist & Winblad, 1999). Alzheimer patients show a major decline in learning new information. Next to anterograde amnesia, they also suffer from retrograde amnesia which is most severe for the more recent memories and the least severe for remote memory (Sadek et al., 2004). Remote memory is not located in the medial temporal lobe but in other brain areas such as the temporal, parietal, and frontal association areas (Sadek et al., 2004). These latter brain areas are affected in a later stage of Alzheimer's disease (Braak & Braak, 1991). In other words, consolidated information becomes independent of the medial temporal lobe (Gilboa et al., 2005). Of note is though that irrespective of the type of episodic memory (recent or remote), the extent of damage to the medial temporal lobe determines the extent of impairment in episodic memory (Gilboa et al., 2005). Also the results of other studies confirm the strong relationship between the medial temporal lobe and episodic memory (Grön & Riepe, 2004). The hippocampus, situated in the medial temporal lobe, shows a high correlation with episodic recognition memory. The medial temporal lobe is also involved in episodic encoding but only in cooperation with other brain areas such as the prefrontal cortex (Rémy et al., 2005). The cooperation between the hippocampus and the prefrontal cortex is reflected in one of the specific functional circuits.

In sum, one of the most prominent clinical symptoms in Alzheimer's disease is an impairment in episodic memory. There is, however, ample evidence that also executive functions are affected in Alzheimer's disease which underscore the functional relationship between the hippocampus (episodic memory) and the prefrontal cortex (executive functions). In other words, the prefrontal cortex is involved in episodic memory processes and the hippocampus in executive functions. An example of a task in which both brain regions plays a role in category fluency.

Other cognitive functions that decline in Alzheimer's disease
Executive functions and episodic memory are not the only cognitive functions that decline in Alzheimer's disease. Besides the neuropathology in brain areas that play a role in the functional circuits described here, also cortico-cortical pathways ('cortical' circuits) connecting association areas of the temporal, prefrontal and parietal lobe are vulnerable but, as described earlier with respect to remote memory, in a later stage. The neuropathology in these areas is responsible for more extensive cognitive impairment that exceeds executive functions and episodic memory (Hof & Morrison, 2004). Impairment is observed in semantic memory (Perry, Watson, & Hodges, 2000), visuospatial functions (Lineweaver, Salmon, Bondi, Corey-Bloom, 2005), language (Kirschner & Bakar, 1995) and the performance of motor activity, reflected in ideomotor apraxia (Kato et al., 2001).

3.3.1 Subcortical ischemic vascular dementia

Within the classification 'vascular dementia', the broadly defined category subcortical ischemic vascular dementia (SIVD) is considered the main cause of vascular cognitive deterioration and dementia (Andin, Gustafson, Passant, & Brun, 2005; Román et al., 2002).

Specific functional circuits
Fronto-subcortical circuits, among which the frontostriatal circuit, are most vulnerable for subcortical white matter lesions and focal lacunar infarcts (Pugh & Lipsitz, 2002). Lacunar infarcts have been observed in the striatum (Kim, Ramachandran, Parisi, & Collins, 1981). Next to a deterioration in motor activity (Elsinger et al., 2003) and cognitive functions, the sensitivity of the frontostriatal system for white matter lesions contributes to depression (O'Brien, Perry, Barber, Gholkar, & Thomas, 2000). This latter point has also been discussed with respect to apathy in Alzheimer's disease.

Atrophy of the hippocampus has been observed in vascular dementia (Bowler, 2002). However, in comparison with other brain areas, the atrophy of the hippocampus is not strongly related to white matter lesions. This is remarkable since the hippocampus is sensitive for a decrease in vascularization (Du et al., 2005). One explanation for this finding might be that cortical areas other than the hippocampus have more prominent subcortical connections which are interrupted by white matter lesions (de-afferentiation) (Du et al., 2005). The hippocampus has less subcortical connections and will therefore be less vulnerable for de-afferentiation. Compared to the hippocampus, the entorhinal cortex has more subcortical connections and will therefore be more affected by white matter lesions. In terms of specific functional circuits, the vulnerability for white matter lesions of the entorhinal cortex implies a decline in the communication between the hippocampus and the prefrontal cortex. A reduced functioning of the prefrontal-hippocampal circuit has also been described in Alzheimer's disease (see figure 2). Of note is that in one study atrophy of the hippocampus was positively related to white matter lesions (den Heijer et al., 2005). This finding can be explained by a correlation that has been found between a low diastolic blood pressure in persons who used anti-hypertensive drugs, atrophy of the hippocampus and white matter lesions. Low blood pressure could be the cause of hippocampal atrophy because the blood vessels, affected by hypertension for many years, are permanently damaged and not able to dilate anymore (den Heijer et al., 2005).

Taken together, the frontostriatal circuit is one of the specific functional circuits that is directly affected by vascular pathology. Also the communication between the hippocampus and the prefrontal cortex declines in vascular dementia by both an indirect (damage of the entorhinal cortex) and a direct way (atrophy of the hippocampus).

The aspecific circuit

Compared to Alzheimer's disease, neuronal loss in brain stem areas are less pronounced in vascular dementia (Yang, Beyreuther, & Schmitt, 1999). In contrast, the cholinergic system, with its origin in the basal forebrain (NBM), is affected in vascular dementia (Román & Kalaria., 2005). As mentioned earlier, the prefrontal cortex, one of the final cortical regions of the ARAS, is strongly involved in vascular dementia because of its vulnerability for white matter lesions and its functional relationship with subcortical areas.

Executive functions and episodic memory

Executive functions

It is quite logical that due to the involvement of fronto-subcortical circuits in vascular dementia, patients with vascular dementia primarily show a decline in executive functions (Pugh & Lipsitz, 2002). The consequence is, among other things, a reduction in psychomotor speed, an impairment in working memory, and an impairment in attention (Román et al., 2002). As mentioned in the section 'Functional circuits in cortical versus subcortical dementia', fronto-subcortical circuits, among which the frontostriatal circuit, are responsible for behavioural disturbances related to executive functions such as a lack of motivation, resulting in apathy (Román et al., 2002). Also opposite reactions such as disinhibited behaviour and impulsivity are frequently observed in vascular dementia (Román et al., 2002). Importantly, interruption of the fronto-subcortical circuits also causes severe disturbances in motor activity, among which disturbances in gait, which resembles gait in Parkinson's disease (Román et al., 2002). For further reading about gait in subcortical ischemic vascular dementia, see chapter 5.

Episodic memory

Episodic memory such as cued recall and recognition memory would remain relatively intact in vascular dementia (Pugh & Lipsitz, 2002). Active retrieval from memory may be impaired but the main cognitive characteristic of subcortical ischemic vascular dementia is 'forgetfulness' (Román et al., 2002). The explanation is that patients with subcortical lesions (as in subcortical ischemic vascular dementia) can still encode and store the information (cortical activities) but are less able to actively retrieve the information from the memory store. Consequently, spontaneous memory shows impairment. However, by providing a cue, for example a recognition-condition, the patient performs much better. If the information has not been properly encoded, as is the case in patients with a cortical lesion, providing a cue is much less effective.

Taken together, in contrast to Alzheimer's disease, executive dysfunctions are the most prominent clinical symptoms of subcortical ischemic vascular dementia. With respect to memory, patients with vascular dementia rather suffer from forgetfulness than from amnesia.

3.3.2 Frontotemporal dementia

Frontotemporal dementia is traditionally divided into three clinical subtypes: the 'frontal variant', the 'temporal variant' and 'progressive non-fluent aphasia' (Hodges, 2001). Within the scope of this chapter only the first two subtypes will be discussed.

3.3.3 'Frontal variant' of frontotemporal dementia

Specific functional circuits

In the 'frontal variant' of frontotemporal dementia, the frontostriatal system is strongly affected (Panegyres, 2004). Compared to Alzheimer's disease, a reduced vascularization has been observed in the anterior cingulate cortex (Varrone et al., 2002). Moreover, the dopaminergic nigrostriatal system is affected (Rinne et al., 2002) and the hippocampus shows a reduced metabolism (Franchesi et al., 2005). As mentioned with respect to other subtypes of dementia, a dysfunction of the anterior cingulate cortex and the hippocampus expresses itself in disinhibited behaviour whereas a clinical manifestation of a prefrontal dysfunction is apathy (Franchesi et al., 2005).

The aspecific functional circuit

In comparison with Alzheimer's disease, not all brain stem areas are affected in the frontal variant of frontotemporal dementia (Yang & Schmitt, 2001). Obviously, the prefrontal cortex, the final cortical area of the ARAS, is affected (Garraux et al., 1999).

Executive functions and episodic memory

Executive functions

Three out of the four executive functions (Lezak, 1995), i.e., volition (taking initiatives, goal setting and motivation), purposive action and self-regulation, and effective performance, are impaired in the frontal variant of frontotemporal dementia (Duke & Kaszniak, 2000). There is some empirical evidence for an impairment in planning and for an impairment in executing motor activity in the appropriate sequence (Duke & Kaszniak, 2000). For further details on executive functions, please see the section in which these patients are compared to Alzheimer patients.

Disturbances in behavioural and personality are prominent clinical symptoms of frontal frontotemporal dementia (Duke & Kaszniak, 2000). More specifically, the frontal variant of frontotemporal dementia is characterized by disinhibited behaviour, reduced impulse control, anti-social behaviour, stereotypical behaviour, compulsiveness, Klüver-Bucy syndrome (sexual overactivity, hyperorality), and apathy (Hodges, 2001). As described earlier, this latter symptom might be due to an impairment in 'volition'. These opposite behavioural symptoms have also been described in Alzheimer's disease and vascular dementia. Patients with the frontal variant of frontotemporal dementia become very dependent of the environment because their intern record declines progressively.

In sum, disturbances in behaviour and personality as well as executive dysfunctions are early clinical symptoms of the 'frontal variant' of frontotemporal dementia.

Episodic memory

Not in the initial stages but during the course of the disease more problems in episodic memory occur, such as learning and recall of new information (anterograde amnesia); recognition is better than active retrieval from memory (Hodges, 2001). Also an impairment in remote memory occurs (Hodges, 2001) which, as mentioned before, is located in among others, the frontal association areas (Sadek et al., 2004). Other cognitive functions, such as orientation, recent memory, visuospatial abilities, naming, word-picture matching and the performance of semantic tasks, remain relatively intact (Hodges, 2001).

3.3.4 'Temporal variant' of frontotemporal dementia

Specific functional circuits
Brain areas that play a role in the specific functional circuits and are affected in the 'temporal variant' of frontotemporal dementia are the prefrontal cortex (Seeley et al., 2005), the hippocampus (van de Pol et al., 2005), and the parahippocampal gyrus (Chan et al., 2001; Davies, Graham, Xuereb, Williams, & Hodges, 2004). Atrophy of the hippocampus is not a consistent finding, though (Hodges, 2001). Studies examining neuropathology in other areas of the specific functional circuits such as the cerebellum, the anterior cingulate cortex, and the substantia nigra could not be found. These findings imply that two specific functional circuits may be vulnerable in this variant of frontotemporal dementia: the frontohippocampal circuit and the parietohippocampal circuit.

The aspecific functional circuit
As far as we know, the relationship between brain stem areas, such as the locus coeruleus, the dorsal raphe nucleus, the pedunculopontine tegmental nucleus, and this subtype of frontotemporal dementia has not been examined.

Executive functions and episodic memory

Executive functions
In view of the location of the neuropathology, one can understand that executive functions are relatively preserved in patients with the temporal variant of fronto-temporal dementia. The relative preservation of executive functions might explain why these patients function well in daily life, particularly in their own environment (Hodges, 2001).

Episodic and semantic memory
The core neuropathology in the temporal variant of frontotemporal dementia is located in the anterior lateral temporal lobe (Seeley et al., 2005). Consequently, patient's episodic memory remains relative intact. The temporal variant of fronto-temporal dementia is also called 'semantic dementia' (Davies et al., 2004), because semantic memory is primarily affected, rather than episodic memory. The clinical manifestation of an impairment in semantic memory is a decrease in category fluency (also observed in the frontal variant of frontotemporal dementia and Alzheimer's disease!) with a preservation of only broad categories, an impairment in vocabulary, a decrease in understanding infrequent words, and difficulty in reading and spelling irregular words. Semantic knowledge, necessary to pronounce difficult, infrequent words, is lacking (Hodges, 2001). Phonology and syntax remain

intact. One explanation is that the prefrontal cortex is involved in phonology (Gold, Balota, Kirchhoff, & Buckner, 2005). Remote memory shows an impairment in semantic dementia (Hodges, 2001), which might be due to the neuropathology located in the lateral areas of the temporal lobe (Sadek et al., 2004).

Early stage frontotemporal dementia	
'Frontal variant'	**'Temporal variant'**
Disturbed	**Disturbed**
Behaviour and personality	**Behaviour and personality**
Disinhibited behaviour	Dependent on which hemisphere is affected
Reduced impulse control	
Anti-social behaviour	
Stereotypic behaviour	
Compulsive behaviour	
Klüver-Bucy syndrome	
Apathy	
Cognition	**Cognition**
Reduced executive functions	Reduced semantic memory
Anterograde amnesia	Reduced word fluency
Reduced 'remote memory'	Reduced comprehension infrequent words
Decrease in spontaneous speech	Decline in vocabulary
	Problems with spelling/reading infrequent words
	Decrease in remote memory
Relatively spared	**Relatively spared**
Cognition	**Cognition**
Visuospatial abilities	Executive functions
Orientation	Visuoconstructive functions
Recent memory	Episodic memory
Naming	Phonology and syntax
Matching words and pictures	Orientation
Semantic tasks	

Table 3. Cognitive differences between the 'frontal variant' and 'temporal variant' of early stage frontotemporal dementia (Hodges, 2001).

Cognitive differences between the frontal and temporal variant of frontotemporal dementia

As table 3 shows, in patients with the frontal variant of frontotemporal dementia disturbances in behaviour and personality are characteristic from disease onset, together with an impairment in executive functions, and followed by an impairment in episodic memory functions in a later stage. In the temporal variant of frontotemporal dementia, it depends on which hemisphere is most affected: left hemisphere patients primarily show a decline in semantic knowledge, right hemisphere patients primarily show emotional and behavioural disturbances (Seeley et al., 2005).

'Temporal variant' of frontotemporal dementia in the left and right hemisphere
A division is possible between the temporal variant affecting the right or left hemisphere (Edwards-Lee et al., 1997; Seeley et al., 2005). Patients with a temporal variant in the left hemisphere show primarily a decline in semantic knowledge, reflected in anomia, word finding difficulties, and repetitive speech (Seeley et al., 2005). Of note is that aphasia has also been observed in bilateral neuropathology and neuropathology in the right hemisphere (Edwards-Lee et al., 1997).

Frontotemporal dementia – Temporal variant

Right hemisphere	Left hemisphere
Early stage	**Early stage**
Behavioural/personality disturbances	Decline in semantic knowledge
Socially clumsy	Executive functions intact
Agitated/irritated	Visuoconstructive abilities intact
Apathy	Normal social behaviour
Alcohol abuse	
Loss of libido	
Insomnia	
Verbal and physical threats	
Depression	Depression
Lack of insight	Anhedonia
Denial of disease	Feelings of worthlessness
Eccentric behaviour	Crying
Strange dressing habits	
Bad personal hygiene	
Compulsions	
Later stage	**Later stage**
Decline in semantic knowledge	Behavioural/personality symptoms
Problems with recognizing faces	Problems with recognizing faces

Table 4. Cognitive and psychiatric differences between a right and left hemisphere lesion in patients with semantic dementia (Edwards-Lee et al., 1997).

Although behavioural, personality and psychiatric disturbances occur in all patients irrespective of the location, behavioural and personality problems occur more frequently in right hemisphere patients in the initial stage of the disease (Seeley et al., 2005). Right hemisphere patients behave socially clumsy, agitated and irritated. Verbal and physical threats occur frequently in these patients. In contrast, left hemisphere patients are socially pleasant and show normal social behaviour. Depression occurs in both patient groups but the nature of the depression differs. In right hemisphere patients the depression expresses itself in a lack of insight and denial of the disease, eccentric behaviour among which inconsistency in dressing (e.g., wearing socks that do not match) and bad personal hygiene. Moreover, right hemisphere patients may feel visually attracted to things which may even lead to shoplifting (Edwards-Lee et al., 1997).

In left hemisphere patients, the depression has a more classical nature with anhedonia, feelings of worthlessness and crying (see table 4). During the course of the disease, behavioural, personality, and psychiatric symptoms occur in both subtypes (Seeley et al., 2005). Moreover, in a later stage, both groups experience problems with recognizing faces (Seeley et al., 2005) (see table 4).

Cognitive differences between frontotemporal dementia and Alzheimer's disease
The extent to which cognitive flexibility, attention, and working memory impair, appears not to differ significantly between both subtypes of dementia (Duke & Kaszniak, 2000). Table 5 provides an overview of the similarities and differences in executive functions as indicated by Duke and Kaszniak (2000) between the 'frontal variant' of frontotemporal dementia and Alzheimer's disease. The performance on the Wisconsin Card Sorting Test, a task requiring set-shifting, declines more in the frontal variant of frontotemporal dementia than in Alzheimer's disease (Duke & Kaszniak, 2000). An impairment in disease insight is also typical for the frontal variant of frontotemporal dementia and is possibly more prominent compared to Alzheimer's disease (Duke & Kaszniak, 2000). The results from a study in which the diagnosis of frontotemporal dementia and Alzheimer's disease was confirmed by autopsy showed that patients with frontotemporal dementia performed worse on category and letter fluency than patients with Alzheimer's disease but better on episodic memory tests and visuoconstructive tasks like drawing a clock (Rascovsky et al., 2002). The impaired performance on word fluency might be associated with a dysfunction of the frontal lobe, characteristic for frontotemporal dementia, and the impairment in episodic memory and visuoconstructive disturbances might be caused by a dysfunction of the medial temporal and parietal lobe, typical for Alzheimer's disease.

Disturbances in executive functions	AD	FTD
'Volition'		
Taking initiative (apathy or disinhibition)	!	++
Formulate goals	+	++
Motivation	+	++
Planning/Attention	+	+?
Purposive action/self-regulation		
Production	+	!(!)
Cognitive flexibility	+	+
Set-shifting	+	++
Working memory	+	+
Efficient execution of performances/self-monitoring		
Extent of disease awareness	+	++*

Table 5. Disturbances in executive functions in Alzheimer's disease (AD) and frontotemporal dementia (FTD); + = affected; ++ = more affected; +?: conflicting results with respect to planning; ++*: much earlier present in FTD compared to AD; +(+): a larger disturbance in FTD compared to Alzheimer's disease has not been observed in every study.

Even if all three subtypes of frontotemporal dementia are combined into one group, called frontotemporal lobar degeneration, the differences in cognition and behaviour with Alzheimer's disease remain (Rosen et al., 2002). Memory problems and perceptual disturbances occur much more frequently in Alzheimer's disease than in frontotemporal lobar degeneration; this latter group of patients performs worse on 'frontal' tasks and shows more social and personality disturbances.

Cognitive differences between Alzheimer's disease and subcortical ischemic vascular dementia

It is interesting to compare cognitive dysfunction in Alzheimer's disease with cognitive dysfunction in subcortical ischemic vascular dementia. Compared to vascular dementia, Alzheimer patients perform worse on tasks that appeal to episodic memory such as story recall, and recall and recognition of a list of words (Traykov et al., 2005) (table 6). Alzheimer patients showed more perseverations in category fluency, whereas patients with vascular dementia show perseverations on more 'frontal' tasks such as the Wisconsin Card Sorting task. The Wisconsin Card Sorting task is vulnerable for an impairment in set-shifting, an executive function that appeals to the frontostriatal circuits (Traykov et al., 2005).

The results of a recent study show that drawing certain elements of a clock, such as the appropriate positioning of the hands, is worse in patients with vascular dementia than in patients with Alzheimer's disease (Heinik, Solomesh, Raikher, & Lin, 2002). An explanation might be that drawing the hands of a clock shows a strong relationship with visuospatial capacities and executive functions (Heinik et al., 2002) (table 6). In another recent study the cognitive profile of patients with Alzheimer's disease and vascular dementia was compared to the cognitive profile of older persons without dementia (Graham, Emery, & Hodges, 2004). The results show that, compared to patients with vascular dementia and older persons without dementia, Alzheimer patients perform worse on episodic memory tasks (direct recall, delayed recall and recognition) while patients with vascular dementia perform worse on tasks appealing to executive functions and attention such as letter fluency. Letter fluency is a word fluency task in which one has to name as many words as possible, starting with a specific letter, for example F, A and S. Semantic memory is more affected in vascular dementia (Graham et al., 2004).

In comparison with older persons without dementia, both subtypes of dementia show a similar impairment in naming, attention/short-term memory, comprehension, problem solving capacity, and word fluency.

Cognitive functions	Alzheimer's disease	Subcortical ischemic vascular dementia
Episodic memory		
Story recall	++	+
Recall of list of words	++	+
Recognition of learned words	+	
Semantic memory		+
Word fluency (category fluency)		
Total score	+	+
Perseverations	+	
Word fluency (letter fluency)		+
Executive functions		
WCST Categories	+	+
WCST Perseverations	+	++
Visuospatial functions (clock drawing hands)		+

Table 6. Cognitive differences between Alzheimer's disease and vascular dementia. +: affect-ted; ++ more prominent affected.

3.4 Summary

Each paragraph will start with a brief summary of the brain areas that belong to the specific circuits and the aspecific circuit and are affected in Alzheimer's disease, subcortical ischemic vascular, and the frontal and temporal variant of frontotemporal dementia, followed by the influence of these disorders on executive functions and episodic memory. Subsequently, the main differences between the three major subtypes of dementia, i.e., Alzheimer's disease, vascular dementia, and frontotemporal dementia, are presented.

3.4.1 Alzheimer's disease

Table 7 presents the brain areas that are affected in Alzheimer's disease and play a role in specific functional circuits and in the aspecific functional circuit, the ARAS.

Specific functional circuits	ARAS
Hippocampus	LC
Entorhinal cortex	DRN
Parahippocampal cortex	PPTN
Striatum	NBM
PFC	PFC

Table 7. Brain areas belonging to specific functional circuits and the ARAS (Ascending Reticular Activating System), affected in Alzheimer's disease. LC: locus coeruleus, DRN: dorsal raphe nucleus, PPTN: pedunculopontine tegmental nucleus, NBM: nucleus basalis of Meynert, PFC: prefrontal cortex.

Cognitive decline in Alzheimer's disease
Executive functions. Executive functions such as attention, working memory, abstract thinking, and concept formation are impaired in Alzheimer's disease. A disturbance in 'volition', an executive function that normally reflects taking initiatives, goal setting, and motivation, expresses itself in problems in behaviour and mood such as apathy, depression, hyperactivity, restlessness, and agitation.

Episodic memory. Anterograde and retrograde amnesia is characteristic for Alzheimer's disease. Remote memory is less vulnerable and becomes affected in later stages.

Other cognitive functions. A comprehensive review of all cognitive functions that may decline in Alzheimer's disease is beyond the scope of this chapter. Known cognitive functions that impair in Alzheimer's disease are semantic memory, visuospatial functions, and language.

3.4.2 Subcortical ischemic vascular dementia

Brain areas that belong to specific functional circuits and the ARAS in subcortical ischemic vascular dementia are summarized in table 8.

Specific functional circuits	ARAS
Hippocampus	NBM
Entorhinal cortex	PFC
Striatum	
PFC	

Table 8. Brain areas that are affected in Subcortical Vascular Ischemic Dementia (SIVD) and play a role in specific functional circuits and the ARAS (Ascending Reticular Activating System). NBM: nucleus basalis of Meynert; PFC: prefrontal cortex.

Cognitive decline in subcortical ischemic vascular dementia
Executive functions. In view of the vulnerability of fronto-subcortical circuits for white matter lesions and thus for vascular problems, executive dysfunctions can be anticipated here. Furthermore, cognitive but also behavioural disturbances related to executive functions are observed in this subtype of dementia. The disturbance in fronto-subcortical circuits also causes disturbances in motor activity.

Episodic memory. Patients with this subtype of dementia show 'forgetfulness' instead of amnesia.

3.4.3 Frontal variant of frontotemporal dementia

In the frontal variant of frontotemporal dementia affected brain areas that belong to specific functional circuits and the ARAS, are presented in table 9.

Specific functional circuits	ARAS
Hippocampus	PFC
Anterior cingulate cortex	
PFC	

Table 9. Brain areas that are affected in the frontal variant of frontotemporal dementia and that play a role in specific functional circuits and the ARAS (Ascending Reticular Activating System). PFC: prefrontal cortex.

Cognitive decline in the frontal variant of frontotemporal dementia

Executive functions. The frontal variant of frontotemporal dementia is primarily characterized by cognitive, behavioural, and personality disturbances that are related to executive functions.

Episodic memory functions. An impairment in episodic memory occurs in the later stage of this subtype of dementia.

3.4.4 Temporal variant of frontotemporal dementia

Table 10 presents the brain areas that belong to specific functional circuits and the ARAS and are involved in the temporal variant of frontotemporal dementia.

Specific functional circuits	ARAS
Hippocampus	PFC
Parahippocampal gyrus	
Prefrontal cortex	

Table 10. Brain areas that show neuropathology in the temporal variant of frontotemporal dementia and that play a role in the functioning of specific functional circuits and the ARAS.

Cognitive decline in the temporal variant of frontotemporal dementia

Executive functions. Executive functions are hardly impaired in the temporal variant of frontotemporal dementia, explaining that these patients can function rather independently in daily life.

Episodic and semantic memory. Obviously, impairment in semantic memory is characteristic for this subtype of dementia.

3.4.5 Alzheimer's disease versus frontotemporal dementia

Both disorders show a considerable overlap but the most striking features in frontotemporal dementia are the executive functions-related behavioural and personality disturbances rather than episodic memory impairment which is characteristic for Alzheimer's disease.

3.4.6 Alzheimer's disease versus subcortical ischemic vascular dementia

Overall, there is a considerable overlap in the clinical manifestation of Alzheimer's disease and Subcortical Ischemic Vascular Dementia. The major difference between both disorders is that episodic memory impairment is strongly related to Alzheimer's disease and executive dysfunctions are more strongly associated with Subcortical Ischemic Vascular Dementia. With respect to memory, forgetfulness is observed in patients with Subcortical Ischemic Vascular Dementia whereas amnesia is typical for Alzheimer's disease.

3.5 Questions

1. Describe the difference between cortical and subcortical lesions with respect to memory, language/speech, gross motor activity, behaviour, and mood.
2. Which two specific functional circuits are damaged by the degeneration of the hippocampus in Alzheimer's disease?
3. Is Alzheimer's disease characterized by white matter lesions?
4. Do executive dysfunctions occur in Alzheimer's disease?
5. Is an impairment in category fluency in Alzheimer's disease due to neuropathology in the hippocampus, in the prefrontal cortex, or in both? Please explain.
6. Which specific functional circuits play a role in category fluency and in letter fluency?
7. Can you explain why opposite behaviours like apathy and hyperactivity may occur in Alzheimer's disease?
8. Why is remote memory less vulnerable in Alzheimer's disease?
9. Which specific functional circuit is involved in episodic memory?
10. Why is atrophy of the hippocampus not primarily due to white matter lesions?
11. Which specific functional circuit is disturbed by a degeneration of the entorhinal cortex?
12. Is the ARAS affected in Subcortical Ischemic Vascular Dementia?
13. Why do patients with vascular dementia show primarily a decline in executive functions?
14. Why does episodic memory remain relatively intact in vascular dementia?
15. Can you explain why providing a cue can improve episodic memory performance?
16. Mention three 'variants' of frontotemporal dementia.
17. Which specific functional system is particularly involved in the 'frontal variant' of frontotemporal dementia?
18. Why are disturbances in behaviour and personality prominent clinical symptoms in the frontal variant of frontotemporal dementia?
19. Why do frontal variant frontotemporal dementia patients become dependent of their environment?
20. Could you explain why cognitive functions such as orientation, recent memory, visuospatial abilities, naming, word-picture matching as well as the performance of

semantic tasks remain relatively preserved in the frontal variant of frontotemporal dementia?

21. Which specific functional circuits are vulnerable for the temporal variant of frontotemporal dementia?

22. Which type of memory is particularly impaired in the temporal variant of frontotemporal dementia?

23. Why do patients with the temporal variant of frontotemporal dementia function well in daily life?

24. Which part of the temporal cortex is particularly affected in the temporal variant of frontotemporal dementia?

25. Please indicate the major difference in clinical symptoms between left and right hemisphere semantic dementia.

26. Could you explain why a disturbance in executive functions could be expressed in behavioural and personality disturbances?

27. Could you indicate the major clinical differences between frontotemporal dementia and Alzheimer's disease?

28. Patients with the frontal variant of frontotemporal dementia perform better on episodic memory tasks than patients with Alzheimer's disease. Is the performance on episodic memory unimpaired in the former group?

29. Could you explain why letter fluency is more affected in vascular dementia than in Alzheimer's disease?

30. Please indicate the major difference in cognitive functioning between Alzheimer's disease and vascular dementia.

Chapter 4
Sensory capacities in aging and dementia

4.1 Introduction

In this chapter, the relationship between age and the auditory sensory system, the visual sensory system, the olfactory system (which is closely related to taste), and the somatosensory system, will be discussed. Other topics that will be briefly addressed in this chapter include the relationship between visual and auditory functioning and cognition, and the relationship between sensory function and cognition, reflected in four hypotheses. Disturbances in the various sensory systems have been examined in subtypes of dementia to a much lesser extent; these disturbances will be discussed with respect to Alzheimer's disease, vascular dementia, and frontotemporal dementia.

4.2 Aging

4.2.1 Hearing

The unaffected ear is able to process sound frequencies of 20 Hz – 20 kHz (Yueh, Shapiro, MacLean, & Shekelle, 2003). The frequency for normal speech perception ranges from 250 through 4000 Hz (Frisina & Frisina, 1997; Yueh et al., 2003). The most prevalent hearing loss in aging, with a slowly progressive course, is presbycusis (Cohn, 1999), also called sensorineural hearing loss (Yueh et al., 2003). Sound frequencies between 4000 Hz and 6000 Hz show the largest age effects (Woodruff-Pak, 1997). For patients with presbycusis, hearing is particularly difficult in the presence of background noise (Yueh et al., 2003). An impairment in speech understanding in a noisy environment is partly due to a disturbance in more central auditory structures like the brain stem (Frisina & Frisina, 1997), although presbycusis is assumed to be primarily a peripheral disturbance of the cochlea (Jennings & Jones, 2001). The cochlea shows a hypoperfusion during aging, initiating the release of neurotoxic substances which cause degeneration of the auditory neuroepithelia (Seidman, Ahmad, & Bai, 2002).

Peripheral and central structures may play a role in different aspects of speech understanding. In a longitudinal study, pure tone hearing threshold, speech reception threshold and speech discrimination scores were among the dependent variables that were examined in healthy elderly people with a normal mental status. Assessment took place each year, during a period of 5 years (Enrietto, Jacobsen, & Baloh, 1999). Pure tone hearing threshold is the lowest intensity at which a tone can be perceived. The speech reception threshold was determined by the score at which the participants repeated correctly 50% of two-vowel words like hotdog. The speech discrimination score is the capacity to discriminate between phonetically related words. The results show a progressive increase in pure tone hearing threshold and speech reception threshold and a decrease in speech discrimination. The authors suggest that aging affects both the peripheral and the central auditory systems. Degeneration of the peripheral auditory system such as a loss of neurons in the cochlea could be responsible for the observed increase in pure tone hearing threshold whereas the decline in speech discrimination could be due to disturbances in the central auditory system (Enrietto et al., 1999; Jennings & Jones, 2001).

Also the relationship between hearing and (instrumental) activities of daily life (IADL), independent of physical and cognitive status, has been examined (Keller, Morton, Thomas, & Potter, 1999). The participants were frail elderly. The results show that hearing loss negatively influenced particularly IADL in comparison to activities of daily life (ADL). IADL include for example shopping and it is not illogical that hearing is more involved in these types of activity.

Taken together, hearing is particularly impaired with respect to high frequencies (4000 Hz and 6000 Hz). Disturbances in the central auditory system are responsible for a decrease in speech understanding in a noisy environment and for a decrease in speech discrimination. A decline in the peripheral auditory system causes an increase in pure tone hearing threshold. Importantly, hearing loss has a negative influence on IADL.

4.2.2 Vision

Vision problems occur in 10%-13% of elderly people above 65 years of age who still live at home; this percentage is higher (27%) for elderly people above 85 years of age (Keller et al., 1999). A visual disorder that occurs frequently in the aged population is presbyopia (Strenk et al., 1999). Presbyopia implies, among others, an increase in lens thickness, a decrease in accommodation, and yellowing of the lens. The vision of elderly people is reduced when the lightening is bad (Jackson, Owsley, & McGwin, 1999). Most vision impairments are due to disorders like macular degeneration, cataract, glaucoma and diabetic retinopathy (Corbin & Eastwood, 1986).

Importantly, a reduction in vision capacity has a strong influence on ADL, irrespective of the level of subjects' cognitive functioning (Keller et al., 1999). Elderly people with vision impairments have an increased risk for falls, hip fractures, physical complaints, and depression. Moreover, they need to rely more on the help of other people (Keller et al., 1999). Vision impairment might even enhance mortality (Thompson, Gibson, & Jagger, 1989).

Interestingly, specific visual functions such as the perception of the colours blue, yellow and white as well as the estimation of the (spatial) distance between two stimuli hardly show an age-related decline (Enoch, Werner, Haegerstrom-Portnoy, Lakshminarayanan, & Rynders, 1999). Similarly, elderly people are well able to judge whether an object is on one line with other objects (Enoch et al., 1999), a task that also appeals to the subjects' visuospatial capacity. These capacities are important for object recognition. However, the perception of the moment an object starts to move (movement threshold) does show an age effect (Trick & Silverman, 1991), but may also be due to glaucoma (Nusbaum, 1999).

In sum, age increases the movement threshold but appears to have no effect on colour perception and visuospatial capacity. Vision problems have a strong effect on ADL, physical condition, and mood.

4.2.3 Smell

In the USA, 62.5% of older persons with an age ranging from 80-97 years of age showed an impairment in olfaction (Murphy et al., 2002). Olfaction is divided into various different functions among which: olfactory threshold (lowest concentration at which an odour can be perceived), odour identification, and odour discrimination (Kovács, Cairns, & Lantos, 2004). Olfactory threshold is associated with the peripheral olfactory system whereas odour identification and odour discrimination appeal to cognitive functioning in which the central olfactory system (secondary and tertiary areas) is more involved (Koss, Weiffenbach, Haxby, & Friedland, 1988; Kovács, 2004).

Particularly odour identification shows an age effect (Kovács, 2004). Women perform better on odour identification tasks than men (Kovács, 2004), a difference that disappears in the oldest age group (85-90 years) (Larsson, Nilsson, Olofsson, & Nordin, 2004). In this latter study it was examined which cognitive functions (speed of information processing, executive functions, and semantic memory measured by verbal fluency and vocabulary) contribute to odour identification. Cognitive functions that appear to play a role in odour identification are cognitive speed and vocabulary (Larsson et al., 2004). Executive functions appeared to be unrelated to odour identification. The results further showed that the more education, the more odours could be identified. Discussing the relationship between cognition and odour identification is an invitation to briefly discuss the cortical areas that are involved in olfaction.

One fMRI-study with young and elderly people examined in which cortical areas olfactory stimulation provokes activity and to what extent (Cerf-Ducastel & Murphy, 2003). In that study, the odourants were dissolved in water and subsequently tasted by the subjects; this procedure closely resembles the role of olfaction during eating (Cerf-Ducastel & Murphy, 2003).

Cortical areas involved in olfaction
Piriform cortex
Entorhinal cortex
Amygdala
Hippocampus
Insular lobe
Cerebellum

Table 1. Cortical areas, activated during olfaction

The results show that intensity perception and identification of odours were reduced in older subjects compared to younger subjects. With respect to the cortical areas, activation was observed in the piriform cortex, amygdalar region and entorhinal cortex, areas to which the olfactory bulb primarily projects. These primary olfactory areas project to the orbitofrontal cortex. Moreover, activation has been observed in the insular lobe, hippocampus, and cerebellum (see table 1 and figure 1)

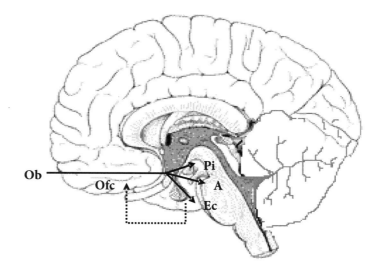

Figure 1. Projection of the olfactory bulb (Ob) to the piriform cortex (Pi), amygdalar region (A), and entorhinal cortex (Ec). These primary olfactory areas project to the orbitofrontal cortex (Ofc) (dotted line).

Results from another fMRI study show that next to the above mentioned areas, also the thalamus and the hypothalamus play a role in olfactory functioning (Wang, Eslinger, Smith, & Yang, 2005).

Another function of the olfactory system is odour recall (Murphy, Nordin, & Acosta, 1997). Although odour recall is based upon odour identification, the age-related decline in odour recall appears not to be exclusively due to a deterioration in odour identification (Murphy et al., 1997). One of the factors that contribute to a decline in odour recall is a decrease in semantic encoding, i.e., the ability to name the odours correctly (Murphy et al., 1997).

4.2.4 Taste

Taste detection threshold and possible alterations in taste (food tastes different than before) were examined in healthy subjects, divided into young, middle-aged and old, and in subjects with chronic renal failure and cancer (Ng et al., 2004). They suggest that an increased taste detection threshold and a change in the taste itself may reduce food intake. The results show that after the age of 70, an increase in taste detection threshold is observed. In patients with chronic renal failure and in patients with cancer, taste itself is affected by e.g., uremic toxins and chemotherapy, respectively (Ng et al., 2004). In another study, the effects of age on taste recognition were examined in healthy elderly subjects (Fukunaga, Uematsu, & Sugimoto, 2005). They observed a significant increase in taste recognition threshold but also in taste detection threshold. The authors suggest that the decrease in taste recognition is more likely due to impaired taste sensation (detection threshold) instead of an impairment in language and memory, cognitive functions that are also involved in taste recognition.

Taken together, age appears to have the strongest influence on odour identification, an olfactory function in which also cognitive speed and vocabulary are involved. Furthermore, odour identification is positively correlated with to the level of education. Correct naming of the odours is important for odour recall. The association between these olfactory functions and higher-level cognitive functions emphasizes the role of cortical areas in olfaction.

An age-related increase in the taste detection threshold is the main cause of an increase in the taste recognition threshold. These findings might seriously affect food intake.

4.2.5 Relationship between a decline in smell, taste, body weight and physical activity

A decline in taste, and more particularly in smell, changes the flavour of food, decreasing food intake, enhancing weight loss and causing anorexia in aging. Flavour is "the sensation that is produced when a substance is placed in the mouth" (Morley, 2001, p. 81).

Importantly, loss of smell and taste may harm the appetite of elderly people. A loss of appetite may reduce the nutritional state and the functioning of the immune system, increasing the risk for other diseases (Schiffman, 2000). Loss of weight might also be one of the consequences (Schiffman, 2000). One way to improve food intake is to intensify the taste and the smell of the food which might strengthen the appetite of the elderly people. Also varying the flavours enhances the chance that at least one of the meals will be taken (Schiffman, 1997). Results show that these food-additives may improve the quality of life (Schiffman, 2000). One should be cautious, however, since an increase in salt or sugar to lower the taste threshold may have adverse effects on the subjects' health (Nusbaum, 1999). Moreover, an increase in the consumption of food with more flavour not necessarily leads to more body weight; its effectiveness may depend on the period the person is exposed to a more flavoured diet (MacIntosh, Morley, & Chapman, 2000).

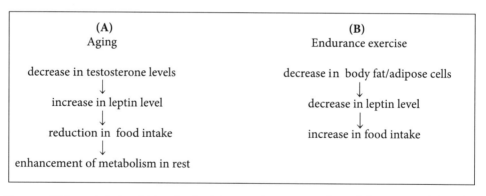

Figure 2. Vicious circle in which aging leads to an enhancement of metabolism in rest (A); endurance exercise will result in an increase in food intake (B).

Next to a decline in taste and smell as a cause for a reduction in food intake, also physiological processes intrinsic to the aging process may be responsible for the reduced food intake (Morley, 2001). Morley (2001) describes the following vicious circle (figure 2): during aging, the testosterone level decreases, causing an increase in leptin, a hormone secreted by adipose cells. The increase in leptin subsequently reduces food intake and enhances the rate of metabolism in rest. Malnutrition may further cause a reduction in muscle mass and muscle strength (MacIntosh et al., 2000) and hence in physical activity. On the other hand, endurance exercise such as bicycling decreases body fat, and hence adipose cells; consequently the level of leptin decreases and food intake increases (for further reading, see Morley, 2001; MacIntosh et al., 2000).

4.2.6 Somatosensory system

Touch

About 25% of the elderly population show a reduction in the detection of tactile stimuli (Kenshalo, 1977). The decrease in aged people to detect tactile stimuli (pressure on the skin) may be due to a decrease in the number of Meissner and Pacini corpuscles (Heft, Cooper, O'Brien, Hemp, & O'Brien, 1996). Aging has no severe effect on free nerve endings but when it has, changes occur in the thick myelinated A-βeta fibres (mechanoreceptors) and much less in A-Delta and C-fibres (Kenshalo, 1986).

Next to peripheral mechanisms, also central mechanisms like fatigue, distraction, and motivation play a role in the tactile sensory detection threshold in aging (Schmidt & Wahren, 1990). The contribution of the peripheral and central nervous system to the tactile sensory detection threshold in elderly people was also examined in another elegant study applying two different two-point discrimination tests (Woodward, 1993). A two-point discrimination test assesses the minimum space between two points, applied simultaneously to the skin, necessary for the subject to perceive two separate points instead of one. The two tests included in that study were: a 'two-point wheel' that produced various depths of skin indentation and a 'gap wheel' that applied a varying gap between two points without losing contact with the skin. The rationale was that changes in the tactile detection threshold that paralleled the various depths of skin indentation (two-point wheel) would support a peripheral sensory mechanism. However, if the tactile detection threshold is not determined by the extent of skin indentation than two-point discrimination would be more dependent on a central sensory mechanism (Woodward, 1993). The results show that age had an effect on both sensory mechanisms. In addition, a relationship was found between skin indentation (two-point wheel) and the level of the tactile detection threshold, in other words, the more skin indentation, the lower the level of tactile detection threshold (Woodward, 1993). The author suggests that factors related to the properties of the skin or changes in the central nervous system such as speed of information processing are responsible for the observed effects.

Apart from speed of information processing, cognitive functions do not play a prominent role in the tactile detection threshold in aging. In one study, a two-point discrimination test was applied to either the index finger or the forearm (Stevens, 1992). The age effect was particularly associated with the tactile detection threshold of the index finger and hardly with the tactile detection threshold of the forearm. In other words, a disturbance in two-point discrimination is primarily caused by changes in the sensory system and not by an age-related decline in memory, attention, and fatigue; otherwise there would be no difference in the tactile detection threshold between the finger and the forearm (Stevens, 1992).

To examine tactile spatial acuity, fine grating domes were applied to the fingertip of older people (Tremblay, Wong, Sanderson, & Coté, 2003). The older participant was requested to indicate the perceived direction of the grooves, i.e., along or across the fingertip. Particularly older persons had difficulty in indicating the direction of the grooves. Importantly, those with a less fine spatial acuity (lower scores on the fine grating domes) performed worse on a test highly demanding for hand and finger movements (the Grooved Pegboard test). In other words, those with impaired tactile spatial acuity showed impaired hand function on a test that really required fine manipulations of the index finger and thumb (Tremblay et al., 2003).

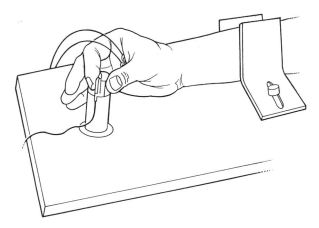

Figure 3. Right arm and digits positioned for measuring pinch force. This arrangement is used for measuring both maximal and submaximal pinch forces. The transducer is aligned with the pads of the index finger and the thumb. Reprinted with permission from Tranganathan, V.K., Siemionow, V., Sahgal, V., & Yue, G.H. (2001). Effects of aging on hand function. Journal of the American Geriatrics Society, 49(11), 1478-1484. Blackwell Science Inc, Malden, USA.

Also in a 3-years longitudinal study with healthy community-dwelling elderly people, subjects' tactile capacity, measured by e.g., tactile recognition of every-day objects, decreased (Desrosiers, Hébert, Bravo, & Rochette, 1999). Of note is that in this study the functioning of the whole upper extremity decreased during this period. Interestingly, those who performed the worst at baseline were the subjects who died during the study; probably their health was more affected and their ADL) more reduced than those who performed better at baseline (Desrosiers et al., 1999). Other studies confirm an age-related decrease in the ability to discriminate between two stimuli that are applied simultaneously to the skin (two-point discrimination) and, in addition, a decrease in grip strength, pinch force (figure 3), pinch posture (figure 4), and speed to relocate (Ranganathan, Siemionow, Sahgal, & Yue, 2001a). They emphasize again that a reduction in hand function has a negative effect on the quality of life of older persons.

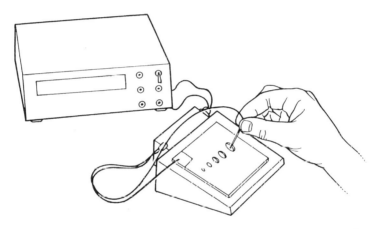

Figure 4. Arrangement for testing the ability to maintain a steady pinch posture (precision pinch steadiness). A metal probe was inserted by subjects into holes of progressively decreasing diameters and held steady for 15 seconds. Reprinted with permission from Tranganathan, V.K., Siemionow, V., Sahgal, V., & Yue, G.H. (2001). Idem. Blackwell Science Inc, Malden, USA.

As far as the author knows, a relationship between tactile information processing of the feet, walking and aging has not been examined so far.

Appropriate processing of oral tactile information is essential for older persons to adapt to age-related changes in eating movements (Wohlert, 1996). The lips contain, among others, many Meissner corpuscles and free nerve endings. Wohlert (1996) examined the tactile perception of spatial stimuli by the upper and lower lip of young and older people by grating orientation discrimination (Wohlert, 1996). For this purpose, a plastic dome consisting of a grating with bars and grooves was used (see figure 5).

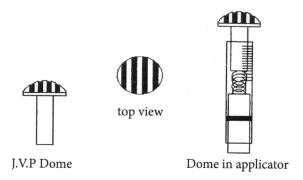

J.V.P Dome   Dome in applicator

Figure 5. To assess the perception of tactile stimuli by the lips, gratings, cut into domes, are pressed against the lip surface. Reprinted with permission from Wohlert, A.B., 1996. Tactile Perception and Spatial Stimuli on the Lip Surface by Young AND Older Adults. Journal of Speech, Language and Hearing Research, 39 (6), 1191/1198. American Speech-Language-Hearing Association, Rockville, USA.

The participants had to indicate whether the bars were in a horizontal or vertical position on the left and right side of the upper and lower lip. The results show that the acuity of the spatial perception declines with age. No differences in tactile perception were observed between the upper and lower lip and between the left and right side of the lips. These results could be explained by a significant decrease in the number of Meissner corpuscles; in other words the mechanism underlying the observed effects is of a peripheral origin (Wohlert, 1996).

In sum, the age-related decline in the detection of tactile stimuli occurs in the upper extremity, particularly in the hand and fingers, probably due to a decrease in the number of Meissner and Pacini corpuscles. Apart from processing speed, cognition appears not to play a role in the tactile detection threshold. A decrease in detecting tactile stimuli by the hand has serious consequences for the recognition of every-day objects which may partly explain the decrease in ADL and the decline in quality of life. The decrease in the perception of tactile stimuli by the lips may negatively influence eating.

Static and dynamic joint-position sense
It is known that a decline in joint-position sense in older people negatively influences gait (Hurley, Rees, & Newham, 1998), enhances a reduction in postural stability (Lord, Clark, & Webster, 1991) and, hence, the risk for falls (Hurley et al., 1998). Within this scope, studies examining static and dynamic position-sense of the lower limb joints of older people are most important.

Static joint-position sense

With respect to the knee, studies show that people more precisely indicate the joint angle if the knee has to bear full weight (more afferent sensory information from the joint) instead of no weight (Marks, Quinney, & Wessel, 1993).

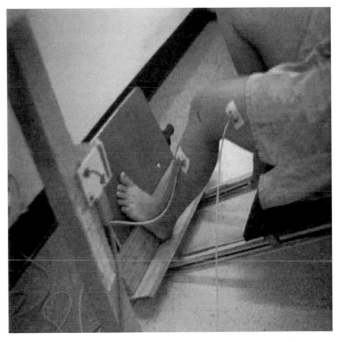

Figure 6. Experimental set-up in the study of Bullock-Saxton et al. (2000). Reprinted with permission from Bullock-Saxton, J.E., Wong, W.J., & Hogan, N.(2001). The influence of age on weight-bearing joint reposition sense of the knee. Experimental Brain Research, 136(3), 400-406. Springer Verlag, New York.

Bullock-Saxton and co-workers (2000) examined the age effect on the joint-position sense of the knee in two conditions: full-weight and partial weight (see figure 6). The latter condition is important since many elderly people can only partially load their knee joint because of e.g., osteoarthritis (Bullock-Saxton, Wong, & Hogan, 2000).

The results show only an age effect in the partial weight condition (Bullock-Saxton et al., 2000). The authors state that in this condition information about the joint-angle is particularly transmitted through muscle receptors and not through joint mechanoreceptors, which mediate proprioceptive information during passive joint movements. Important with respect to older people is that joint-position sense of the knee is further reduced by fatigue (Skinner, Wyatt, Hodgdon, Conard, & Barrack, 1986).

In line with this finding is the important role of muscle strength, particularly of the quadriceps, in proprioception (Hurley et al., 1998). They found that age had no effect on the voluntary activation of the quadriceps but did decrease its strength. The consequences of reduced quadriceps strength include a decrease in joint position-sense, postural stability, and ADL (see figure 7).

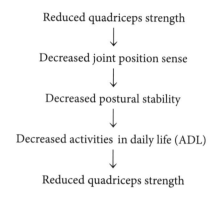

Reduced quadriceps strength
↓
Decreased joint position sense
↓
Decreased postural stability
↓
Decreased activities in daily life (ADL)
↓
Reduced quadriceps strength

Figure 7. A vicious circle initiated by an age-related decrease in quadriceps strength, finally result-ing in a decrease in activities of daily life (ADL)

In sum, weight bearing on the knee highly contributes to the joint-position sense. Partial weight bearing shows an age effect. In other words, muscle strength is im-portant for proprioception; unfortunately, age decreases muscle strength.

Dynamic joint-position sense
Muscle spindles are supposed to play a crucial role in dynamic joint-position sense, i.e., position sense during movement (Verschueren, Brumagne, Swinnen, & Cordo, 2002). In that study, dynamic joint-position sense at the ankle of older people was examined. The participant is sitting behind a computer screen at which three lines, indicating the start position (150 dorsiflexion), the target position (100 plantar flexion) and the final angle (200 plantar flexion) are presented (see figure 8). The ankle, which they could not see, is rotated by a motor. By pressing the index finger and the thumb together, an electrical contact is made. Subsequently, the motor starts to move the ankle. The moment the participant feels that the ankle angle reaches the target position, the participant opens the fingers, an action that interrupts the electrical contact and releases a line on the screen by which the difference between that line and the original line can be calculated.

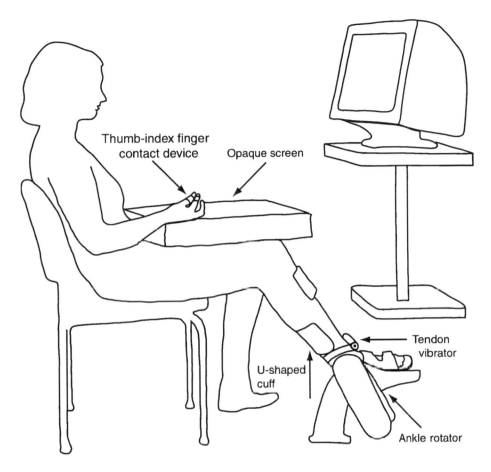

Figure 8. Experimental set-up in the study of Verschueren et al. (2002). Reprinted with permission from Verschueren, S.M.P., Brumagne, S., Swinnen, S., & Cordo, P.J. (2002). The effect of aging on dynamic position sense at the ankle. Behavioural Brain Research, 136(2), 593-603. Elsevier Science, Amsterdam.

The results show that age has an effect on the dynamic position sense. Although the decline was small, the authors suggest that together with other age-related sensory disturbances, the decline in dynamic balance may be sufficient to increase the risk for falls. An alternative explanation might be an age-related decline in divided attention since the subject had to pay attention to both the ankle angle and the movement of the hand (Verschueren et al., 2002).

The cooperation between dynamic joint-position sense and other sensory systems to maintain postural stability may depend on the surface of the floor the person is standing on: firm or foam (Lord et al., 1991). Postural instability in the 'firm' condition is caused by a reduced dynamic joint-position sense together with reduced tactile sensitivity. A decrease in dynamic joint-position sense, together with in a decline in visual acuity, vibration sense, and ankle dorsiflexion strength were associated with postural instability in the 'foam' condition (Lord et al., 1991). In other words, postural stability in the foam condition requires the involvement of much more sensory and motor systems than postural stability in the firm condition.

Another interesting finding is that providing new sensory information during the performance of a task might be beneficial for young people but quite negative for older people. For example, an increase in propriocepsis during a balance task by removal of an apparatus around the ankle that sent disturbing sensory signals, improved balance in young people, but reduced balance in elderly people. Elderly people might not be able to adequately process this changing sensory information (Nusbaum, 1999). In ADL, a reduction in integrating sensory information from different modalities may reflect the often observed decline in walking velocity when the older person has to cross a street.

In sum, a decline in dynamic joint-position sense, together with disturbances in other sensory systems, for example in the visual sensory system, increases the risk for falling, especially when the floor one is standing on, is not firm.

Visual and auditory functioning in relation to cognition

Newson and Kemps (2005) emphasize that little attention has been paid to sensory dysfunctions in aging, a confounding variable that may limit the participation in various types of activity and may influence cognitive functioning. In a recent review, relations between sensory/sensorimotor deficits and cognition in aging have been discussed (Li & Lindenberger, 2002). The findings of this review can be summarized as follows. Cross-sectional correlational analyses showed that hearing and vision, (and balance-gait) explained a high percentage (64.5% – 82.6%) of age-related general intelligence (speed, reasoning, memory, knowledge, and fluency). Longitudinal correlational data-analyses confirm the interdependence between changes in cognition and in sensory functioning, particularly changes in vision. Interesting findings also emerge from experimental studies in which the processing of sensory information was hindered. For example, compared to young adults, older adults had more difficulty recognizing words from sentences that were presented before in a very noisy environment; the same findings were observed when the processing of visual stimuli was hampered. Under these circumstances, particularly long-term memory seems to be vulnerable (Li & Lindenberger, 2002). There are indications that not changes in peripheral but rather in central processing of sensory stimuli are responsible for the decline in cognitive functioning.

Not only a relationship between sensory and cognitive functioning has been established, sensory dysfunction is also predictive for cognitive dysfunction. A study applying cross-sectional regression analyses revealed that hearing and vision predicted particularly speed of processing whereas in longitudinal analyses, also a change in scores on picture naming and verbal fluency was predicted by sensory stimulation (Newson & Kemps, 2005). In a 6-year follow-up study which included elderly of 55 years of age and older, it was observed that a decline in particularly visual but also auditory acuity was predictive for a lower performance on tasks that appeal to visual verbal learning, memory and attention capacities (Valentijn et al., 2005). There appeared to be no relationship between visual and auditory capacity and executive functions. A unique feature of this study was that a relatively small subgroup of these subjects was treated for their sensory deficit (e.g., cataract surgery). The observed lack of beneficial effects of this treatment on cognition might be due to a lack of statistical power (Valentijn et al., 2005).

Taken together, except for executive functions, particularly the visual sensory system but also the auditory sensory system is strongly related to cognitive functioning in aging.

Hypotheses on relationship between sensory function and cognition

Four hypotheses have been described with respect to the relationship between sensory functioning and cognition: 1) the 'sensory deprivation hypothesis', 2) the 'aging induced cognitive load hypothesis of sensory performance', also paraphrased as the 'resource allocation hypothesis', 3) the 'common cause hypothesis' and 4) the 'direct effect of sensory impairment on test performance' hypothesis (Lindenberger & Baltes, 1994; Anstey, Lord, & Williams, 1997; Christensen, Mackinnon, Korten, & Jorm, 2001; Baltes & Lindenberger, 1997; Cabeza, Anderson, Locantore, & McIntosh, 2002; van Boxtel, ten Tusscher, Metsemakers, Willems, & Jolles, 2001). The first two hypotheses concern a direct relationship between sensory and cognitive function.

1) *Sensory deprivation hypothesis.* This hypothesis implies that by a decline in sensory input, the brain is less challenged to exchange information with the environment, consequently will be less stimulated and will therefore be less triggered to process information as effective as possible (Lindenberger & Baltes, 1994; Baltes & Lindenberger, 1997). Findings do not provide much support for the sensory deprivation hypothesis since vocabulary, a cognitive function which is representative for social interaction, did not show a high correlation with sensory functioning (Lindenberger & Baltes, 1994). To support the hypothesis, a decline in vocabulary should go together with a decline in sensory function.

2) *Aging-induced cognitive load hypothesis of sensory performance or resource allocation hypothesis.* This hypothesis implies that during aging relatively simple

sensory tasks become progressively more difficult to perform (Lindenberger & Baltes, 1994; Baltes & Lindenberger, 1997). Since in that case an increasing number of cognitive resources must be activated to perform the sensory tasks, other cognitive processes that should be performed at the same time, may decline (Lindenberger & Baltes, 1994). This hypothesis could also be paraphrased as the 'resource allocation hypothesis': the elderly person has to appeal to more than one source to solve the task satisfactory. For example, elderly persons have to activate both prefrontal cortices to perform a task at the same level as younger people do with only one prefrontal cortex (Cabeza et al., 2002). This and other compensatory mechanisms are further discussed in chapter 6.

3) *Common cause hypothesis.* This hypothesis means that the aging of the central nervous system is the common cause of changes in cognitive and physiological systems (Anstey et al., 1997; Christensen et al., 2001). The finding that lower limb strength, a non-cognitive function, is also correlated with cognitive dysfunction in old age is considered evidence for the 'common cause hypothesis' (Anstey et al., 1997). They indicate that lower limb strength is particularly due to deterioration of motor neurons in the spinal cord which is part of the central nervous system. It has also been suggested that a change in neurotransmitter systems such as the cholinergic system in the motor cortex is responsible for the decrease in limb strength (Anstey et al., 1997). It is known that the cholinergic system also plays a crucial role in learning and memory (Pepeu & Giovannini, 2004).

4) *Direct effect of sensory impairment on test performance hypothesis.* This hypothesis implies that due to sensory impairment, e.g., visual impairment, the older person performs less well on neuropsychological tests appealing to the visual sensory system (van Boxtel et al., 2001).

Conclusions

In sum, a negative consequence of aging is a decline in the processing of sensory stimuli such as auditory, visual, somatosensory, and olfactory stimuli, including taste. Particularly a decrease in smell (olfaction) and taste may lead to malnutrition and finally to a decrease in physical activity. The effect of age on touch (somatosensory system) is noteworthy since a decrease in the processing of tactile stimuli by the upper extremity, particularly the hand and fingers, and the mouth has serious consequences for ADL and food intake, respectively. This sequence of events negatively influences the level of physical activity. An age effect has also been observed for static and dynamic position sense, reducing postural stability and, again, physical activity.

4.3 Alzheimer's disease

4.3.1 Hearing

In an early study, the superior temporal gyrus of 2 Alzheimer patients was examined (Esiri, Pearson, & Powell, 1986). Area 41, the primary auditory cortex, hardly showed neurofibrillary tangles and neuritic plaques. In contrast, in a later postmortem study, senile plaques and neurofibrillary tangles were found in area 41 of 9 Alzheimer patients (Sinha, Hollen, Rodriguez, & Miller, 1993). In that study more severe neuropathology was observed in areas of the central auditory system, i.e., in the medial geniculate body (particularly neurofibrillary tangles), in the inferior colliculus (particularly senile plaques) and in the auditory association cortex (area 22) (neurofibrillary tangles and senile plaques). Degeneration of the medial geniculate body may negatively influence the perception of low and high frequencies. Findings from another study show degeneration of the peripheral auditory system in Alzheimer's disease that did not differ from the degeneration observed in normal aging (Sinha, Saadat, Linthicum, Hollen, & Miller, 1996). In other words, the peripheral auditory system appears not to be further affected by Alzheimer's disease (Sinha et al., 1996).

Taken together, Alzheimer's disease has a specific effect on the central auditory system and shows a hearing impairment for low and high frequencies.

4.3.2 Vision

Obviously, the vision impairments that have been observed during normal aging also occur in Alzheimer's disease. For example, the movement threshold (the moment one sees an object starts to move) is increased in both Alzheimer's disease and normal aging (Trick & Silverman, 1991). They suggest that both with respect to aging and Alzheimer's disease, the impairment in movement threshold is due to a deterioration of the retinocortical pathway that plays a role in visuospatial information processing ('dorsal stream'). However, a more severe impairment in Alzheimer's disease in comparison with normal elderly people concerns the conscious perception of the movement of the object (Silverman, Tran, Zimmerman, & Feldon, 1994). The authors suggest that particularly the medial temporal lobe plays a crucial role in this cognitive function. More specifically, the pathway from the primary visual area (area 17), through the magnocellular part of the lateral geniculate nucleus, to the medial temporal lobe would be responsible (Gilmore, Wenk, Naylor, & Koss, 1994).

In sum, compared to aging, Alzheimer's disease is characterized by an impairment in conscious perception of the movement, a function mediated by the temporal lobe.

4.3.3 Smell and taste

Brain areas which are involved in smell such as the olfactory bulb, the nucleus olfactorius anterior, the prepiriform cortex, the entorhinal cortex, the hippocampus, the amygdala, and the basal forebrain show neuropathology which is characteristic for Alzheimer's disease (Koss et al., 1988; Schiffman, Clark, & Warwick, 1990). In addition, neurotransmitters like acetylcholine are involved in the olfactory system (Koss et al., 1988) and in Alzheimer's disease (Engelborghs & DeDeyn, 1997). The relationship between olfaction and taste has been examined in patients with Alzheimer's disease and with other subtypes of dementia such as vascular dementia (Schiffman et al., 1990). The results show that compared to elderly people without dementia, patients with dementia, irrespective of its etiology, show a decline in the perception of a taste (taste threshold) and in the recognition of an odour. Interestingly, the finding that loss of smell was characteristic for those who had a family history of senile dementia, may imply a genetic component (Schiffman et al., 1990). A decline in the recognition of an odour in Alzheimer's disease has also been found in other studies (Koss et al., 1988; Nusbaum, 1999). Although the results on the involvement of the odour threshold in Alzheimer's disease are equivocal, the olfactory bulb of Alzheimer patients contains more beta-amyloïd than the olfactory bulb of elderly people without dementia (Kovács et al., 1999). They conclude that both the peripheral (olfactory bulb) and central olfactory systems (e.g., hippocampus, amygdala) are affected in Alzheimer's disease and that loss of smell could be an early marker for Alzheimer's disease. Furthermore, it has been suggested that the odour threshold will increase during the course of dementia (Murphy, 1999) and is characteristic for the late stage (Kovács, 2004). Deterioration of odour identification occurs in the early stage of Alzheimer's disease and may even precede a decline in memory (Kovács, 2004). Interestingly, a decrease in these olfactory functions has also been observed in patients with Mild Cognitive Impairment (MCI), a preclinical stage of Alzheimer's disease (Peters et al., 2003). Even subjects who are not cognitively impaired but who are positive for Apolipoprotein E4, showed a higher odour threshold and poorer odour identification (Murphy, 1999).

In sum, odour identification and odour discrimination show a deterioration in Alzheimer's disease (Kovács, 2004). An increase in odour and taste threshold was not a consistent finding.

4.3.4 Somatosensory system

Touch

The primary sensory abilities such as touch remain relatively preserved in Alzheimer's disease (Huff ct al., 1987). Cerebral glucose metabolism is reduced in motor, auditory and visual brain areas but the least in the primary sensomotor areas (Blesa et al., 1996). Indeed, the primary somatosensory areas are relatively preserved in Alzheimer's disease (Braak & Braak, 1991). Particularly secondary somatosensory functions such as stereognosis show a deterioration in Alzheimer's disease (Huff et al., 1987).

Learning by a tactile discrimination task has been examined in Alzheimer patients, patients with Parkinson's disease and older people without dementia (Freedman & Oscar-Berman, 1987). It is argued that tactile discrimination tasks particularly appeal to the parietal lobe. The parietal lobe is affected in Alzheimer's disease (see chapter 1). In contrast, in Parkinson patients particularly the frontal lobe is affected (Dirnberger, Frith, & Jahanshahi, 2005). In the study of Freedman and Oscar-Berman (1987) the patient was sitting behind a table on which two forms, one with the letter 'x' and one with the letter 'o', were placed which could not be seen by the patient (see figure 9).

A coin was hidden under the 'x'. Without seeing the coins the patient had to touch the letters and learn that when he discovered the 'x', he would find the coin. Subsequently, the researcher hide the coin under the 'o' and now the patient had to learn to change his strategy and find the 'o' by touch. The results show that, compared to patients with Parkinson's disease and older persons without dementia, Alzheimer patients performed worse on tactile recognition of the letter 'x'. This finding supports the more pronounced involvement of the parietal lobe in Alzheimer's disease. However, the reduced performance on strategy shifting did not differ between Alzheimer patients and patients with Parkinson's disease, indicating that the frontal lobe is affected in both neurodegenerative diseases (Burton, McKeith, Burn, Williams, & O'Brien, 2004; Harwood et al., 2005).

In sum, stereognosis and tactile recognition decline in Alzheimer's disease.

Static and dynamic joint-position sense
No studies could be found that examined the influence of Alzheimer's disease in static and dynamic joint-position sense.

4.4 Vascular dementia

In contrast to Alzheimer's disease, only a few studies examined the influence of vascular dementia on smell, taste, and somatosensory functioning.

4.4.1 Smell and taste

Taste threshold increased and odour identification declined in patients with vascular dementia (Schiffmann et al., 1990).

4.4.2 Somatosensory

Somatosensory functioning, measured by electrical stimulation of the median nerve and the peroneal nerve (somatosensory evoked potentials: SEPS) was impaired only in those patients who were in an advanced stage and showed subcortical lesions (Tsiptsios et al., 2003).

4.5 Frontotemporal dementia

Similar to vascular dementia, sensory systems are hardly examined in this subtype of dementia.

4.5.1 Hearing

One patient suspected of frontotemporal dementia, showed signs of progressive cortical deafness, i.e., hearing loss for low and middle frequencies, together with progressive articulation problems, in the absence of stroke (Kaga, Nakamura, Takayama, & Momose, 2004).

4.5.2 Somatosensory

Somatosensory functioning, measured by electrical stimulation of the median nerve (SEPS) showed a mild impairment (Rosén, Gustafson, & Risberg, 1993).

4.6 Summary

The clinical consequences of the sensory deficits will be briefly discussed with respect to aging, Alzheimer's disease, vascular dementia, and frontotemporal dementia (table 2).

4.6.1 Aging

An impairment in hearing and vision has a negative influence on the instrumental activities of daily life (IADL); in addition, vision problems increase the risk for falls, physical complaints and depression. Vision problems may even enhance mortality. Another factor that increases the risk for falls is a decline in static and dynamic balance.

Concerning smell, an age-related disturbance in odour identification and in the related odour recall seriously affect food intake. Food intake is also hampered by an increase in the taste detection threshold and the taste recognition threshold since it harms the appetite of the older persons. An important consequence is weight loss. A third factor that influences food intake, and thus enhances weight loss, is the impaired processing of tactile stimuli by the hand, fingers and lips.

Another interesting finding is the relationship between visual and auditory function and cognition. Compared to an impairment in the auditory system, has the visual impairment the highest impact on cognitive function such as long-term memory and attention, but not on executive functions.

4.6.2 Alzheimer's disease

Compared to normal aging, is the peripheral auditory system not further deteriorated in Alzheimer's disease, in contrast to the central auditory system which is severely affected. The impairment in the movement detection threshold and conscious perception of movement in Alzheimer's disease may have serious consequences for IADL, for example in crossing a street with traffic.

Concerning smell and taste, odour identification and odour discrimination decline whereas odour and taste threshold may increase but results are conflicting. Furthermore, with respect to the somatosensory system, tactile recognition, stereognosis, and the fine motor activity of the hand decline in Alzheimer's disease. Similar to aging, the deterioration of the various sensory-motor systems may seriously affect the patients' (I)ADL.

4.6.3 Vascular dementia and frontotemporal dementia

Sensory systems have hardly been examined in these subtypes of dementia. In vascular dementia a decrease in odour identification, an increase in taste threshold, and an impairment in somatosensory functioning have been found. In frontotemporal dementia, impaired hearing for low and middle frequencies has been observed, however only in one patient; also a mild impairment in somatosensory functioning has been identified.

Sensory-motor systems	Aging	Alzheimer's disease	Vascular dementia	Fronto-temporal dementia
Hearing	high frequencies ↓ pure tone thresh. ↑ speech rec. thresh. ↑ speech discrimin. ↓	low/high freq. ↓		low freq. ↓ middle freq. ↓
Vision	presbyopia	consc. percept. mov. ↓		
	movement thresh. ↑	movement thresh. ↑		
Smell	odour identification ↓ odour recall ↓	odour identification ↓ odour discrimination ↓ odour threshold ↑ ?	odour identific. ↓	
Taste	taste detection thresh. ↑ taste recogn. threshold ↑	taste threshold ↑?	taste threshold ↑	
Somato-sensory	touch: hand/fingers ↓ touch: lips ↓ static position sense ↓ dynamic position sense ↓	tactile recognition ↓ stereognosis ↓		

Table 2. The clinical consequences of the sensory deficits with respect to aging, Alzheimer's disease, vascular dementia, and frontotemporal dementia.

4.7 Questions

1. On which sound frequencies does age have the largest effect?
2. Please explain the differences between pure tone hearing threshold, speech perception threshold, and speech discrimination.
3. What is meant by presbyopia?
4. Could you indicate the various consequences of visual impairment in daily life?
5. In which olfactory functions is the central olfactory system involved? And in which olfactory function is the peripheral olfactory system involved?

6. Which cognitive functions are involved in odour identification? Does it surprise you that executive functions are less involved in odour identification?

7. Please mention cortical areas that are involved in olfaction.

8. Could you briefly explain how a decrease in smell and taste could lead to a reduction in the level of physical activity?

9. Please describe an age-related intrinsic physiologic process that may contribute to a reduction in food intake and, consequently, to a reduction in physical activity.

10. Which type of free nerve endings are most vulnerable for aging?

11. What is the relationship between the processing of tactile stimuli by the upper extremity/hand and activities of daily life (ADL)?

12. Has the impairment in the perception of tactile stimuli by the lips a central or a peripheral origin?

13. A negative sequence of events emerges from a reduced strength of the quadriceps, resulting in a decrease in activities of daily life. Please describe this vicious circle.

14. Please explain the effect of visual and auditory impaired function on cognition.

15. Describe four hypotheses concerning the relationship between sensory function and cognition.

16. Does Alzheimer's disease have a negative effect on the auditory function?

17. What effect does Alzheimer's disease have on the perception of an object that moves?

18. Which neurotransmitter system is involved in olfaction in Alzheimer's disease?

19. What is the effect of Alzheimer's disease on taste?

20. What is the effect of Alzheimer's disease on the primary somatosensory areas?

21. Do patients with vascular dementia experience a change in smell and taste?

Chapter 5
Motor activity in aging and dementia

5.1   Introduction

Epidemiological studies have shown a strong but not a causal relationship between the level of physical activity and the level of cognitive functioning (van Gelder et al., 2004; Fratiglioni, Paillard-Borg, & Winblad, 2004). However, results from quite a number of intervention studies show that an increase in aerobic physical activity (e.g., brisk walking) is able to enhance cognition in sedentary healthy older people (Okumiya, et al., 1996; Williams & Lord, 1997; Kramer et al., 1999; Fabre, Chamari, Mucci, Masse-Biron, & Prefaut, 2002). Findings of a recent study show that leisure-time physical activity at midlife protects against dementia (Rovio et al., 2005). Neurobiological, social and mental mechanisms underlying these effects have been excellently reviewed (Colcombe & Kramer, 2003; Churchill et al., 2002).

It is argued that, in contrast to the positive cognitive reaction to increased physical activity, a decrease in physical activity might be associated with a decline in patients' cognitive functioning. More specifically, it is suggested that a decrease in physical activity in neurodegenerative diseases such as dementia might further aggravate the already existing cognitive deterioration. Within this scope, an interesting though not causal relationship is that a decrease in physical activity may precede the onset of dementia (Fratiglioni et al., 2004). In addition, results from a 6-year longitudinal study show that, compared to only cognitive impairment, a preclinical syndrome consisting of a combination of cognitive impairment and motor slowing was the strongest predictor for dementia (Waite et al., 2005).

The finding that cognitive impairment coincides with sensorimotor slowing is not so surprising since the results of a recent PET-study show that cognitive and sensory functioning are both needed for locomotion (Malouin, Richards, Jackson, Dumas, & Doyon, 2003), for example for route finding (see Mulder, Zijlstra, & Geurts, 2002). In other words, in the action of normal skilful and smooth walking the fast integration of motor, perceptual and cognitive processes is embodied. Therefore, focusing on gait is literally focusing on cognition in action.

Interestingly, besides the above-described close relationship between walking and the ability to function independently, upper limb function – more specifically hand motor function – shows a close relationship with ADL. A decline in hand motor function is related to a reduction in the ability to perform functional daily activities, such as moving objects, getting dressed, eating and writing (Shiffman, 1992; Ranganathan, Siemionow, Sahgal, & Yue, 2001a) and hence may affect quality of life (Ranganathan et al., 2001a). The discovery that poor hand motor function is related to a higher level of functional dependence might explain why people with a low hand motor function are more likely to live in a nursing home (Ostwald, Snowdon, Rysavy, Keenan, & Kane, 1989). Not only is hand motor function, especially grip strength, an important predictor of functional disability in older persons, it even appears to be a strong predictor of mortality in, for example, older British men (Ostwald et al., 1989); participants with the lowest hand grip strength ran the greatest risk of mortality.

The above results suggest a close relationship between hand motor function, the ability to function independently, ADL, institutionalization, quality of life, and even mortality. Since cognitive functioning is also related to the ability to function independently, ADL and institutionalization, it might be worthwhile to examine the relationship between cognition and hand motor function in, for example, cognitively intact older people and older people with varying levels of cognitive impairment. The aim of this chapter is to address first the relationship between motor functioning, in particular hand-motor activity and gait, and cognition in aging and dementia. Subsequently, the relationship between physical activity, executive functions and depression will be shortly highlighted, finally followed by the relationship between physical activity, energy expenditure and cognition.

5.2 Hand motor function in aging and dementia; its relationship with Activities of Daily Life

In this section, clinical studies that examined hand motor function in aging and (preclinical) dementia, focusing particularly on Mild Cognitive Impairment (MCI), and Alzheimer's Disease (AD) will be explored. Only one study looked into a possible relationship between hand motor function and vascular dementia (VaD). It will be addressed in a brief section about the contribution of hand motor function assessment to the diagnosis of the various subtypes of dementia. This section concludes with a discussion of the clinical relevance of studying hand motor activity in aging and (preclinical) dementia.

The clinical studies on hand motor function in this section have two key strengths: 1) they all explicitly state the specific diagnosis, e.g., Alzheimer's disease instead of elderly with 'dementia'; and 2) some of them include different groups, viz. older persons without dementia, older people with Mild Cognitive Impairment and Alzheimer patients, thus making it possible to draw a direct comparison between the groups.

5.2.1 Aging

In general, clinical studies reveal an age-related decline in fine hand motor function (e.g., precision grip), in complex hand motor function (e.g., moving blocks from one side to another) and in gross hand motor function (e.g., pinch and grip force) (see table 1 for details of the various studies) (Ranganathan et al., 2001a; Desrosiers, Hébert, Bravo, & Rochette, 1999). A close relationship exists between fine, complex, and gross hand motor function. For example, precision-grip requires a fine-tuned target-related grasping force (Voelcker-Rehage & Alberts, 2005). Older people are less able than younger people to adapt this force to changing targets. Moreover, the finger-pinch force declines in both hands and becomes more variable (Keogh, Morrison, & Barrett, 2006). The latter finding implies that older people use their index finger more and their middle finger less during finger-pinch force tasks. These findings confirm that older people are less able to coordinate the force of individual digits, which is essential for ADL (Shim, Lay, Zatsiorsky, & Latash, 2004). One of the causes of the variable force control is a decline in strength (Sosnoff & Newell, 2006). To compensate for a decline in precision-grip force, older persons may increase their grip force (Gilles & Wing, 2003) by, for example, applying grip patterns that produce more strength (Wong & Whishaw, 2004).

Two examples of everyday fine-motor functional tasks that take more time for older people to perform are pouring milk and removing money from a wallet (Shiffman, 1992). The ability to perform functional tasks is stable until the age of 65 (Smith et al., 1999). After that, a mild decline in fine hand motor function was noticed, with a greater decline after the age of 75. These findings indicate a nonlinear relationship between age and fine hand motor function (Smith et al., 1999). In contrast, grip force (gross hand motor function) declines linearly between the age of 50 and 83, irrespective of gender (Frederiksen et al., 2006). However, in the oldest women the decline in grip strength remains even. Remarkably, a decline in grip strength does not necessarily imply an inability to open medication containers and suchlike (Rahman, Thomas, & Rice, 2002).

Another factor that might influence the relationship between age and task performance is familiarity with the task. In one study, the participants had to perform drawing and writing tasks (Mergl, Tigges, Schröter, Möller, & Hegerl, 1999). In general, the older subjects had a lower mean peak acceleration and exerted less pressure. Also, the older persons' movements were slower and less automated. Notably, the difference between older and younger people was less evident when it came to signing their names, a highly automated task. However, familiarity with a task does not always have a positive effect on performance. A study applying kinematic analysis revealed that, irrespective of age, the duration of a stroke by the

Authors	N	Age (years)	Gender	Measurements	Main findings
Desrosiers et al. (1999)	1*: 360 2*: 264	>60 (mean 73.9)	M: 181; F:179 M: 136; F:128	Gross and fine manual dexterity, global UE performance, UE motor coordination, grip strength, tactile recognition, point discrimination, touch/pressure threshold	Gross and fine manual dexterity ↓, global UE performance ↓, UE motor coordination ↓, grip strength ↓, tactile recognition ↓, point discrimination ↓, touch/pressure threshold ↓
Ranganathan et al. (2001)	Y : 27 O : 28	20-35 65-79	M:13; F:14 M:12; F:16	Handgrip strength, maximum pinch force, steady pinch force, precision pinch posture, speed, point discrimination	Handgrip strength ↓, maximum pinch force ↓, steady pinch force ↓, precision pinch posture ↓, movement speed ↓, two-point discrimination ↓
Voelcker-Rehage & Alberts (2005)	Y: 14 O: 12	19-28 67-75	M:8; F:6 M:6; F:6	Mini Model force transducer for isometric precision grip force	Reduced ability to adjust force to changing targets; force-tracking can be trained but performance of older persons lower than that of younger persons
Keogh et al. (2006)	Y: 13 O: 14	23.8 (±4.7) 75.7 (±2.5)	n.a. n.a.	Assessment of tri-digit finger-pinch force by XTran 250 N S-beam load cell transducer and BC302 117.6 N	Older persons show less control over finger-pinch force, use their index finger more and their middle finger less than younger persons
Shim et al. (2004)	Y: 12 O: 12	26.5 (±3.1) 26.0 (±2.4) 86.7 (±9.6) 78.3 (±2.9)	M:6 F:6 M:6 F: 6	Assessment of maximal and submaximal force of all digits by transducers for fingers and thumb	A decline in digit coordination, necessary for producing combinations of force and moment
Sosnoff & Newell, 2006	Y: 15 O: 33	24.9 (±3.8) 70.9 (±5.6)	M:9; F:6 M:15; F:18	Isometric force assessment of the abduction of the index finger	A strong relationship between the variability in force and strength
Gilles & Wing, 2003	Y: 16 O: 15	18-29 59-70	M:5; F:11 M:6; F: 9	Assessment of grip force during up and down movements, with changes in load force (cylindrical force transducer)	A higher grip force in older persons than in younger persons; adjusting grip force to changes in load force similar in older and younger persons
Wong & Whishaw, 2004	VY: 48 Y: 74 O: 16	5-12 15-63 56-77	M:28; F:20 M:34; F:40 M:5; F:11	Assessment of grasping patterns by grasping beads of various diameters	Older persons showed fewer different grasp patterns than younger persons and selected grasps that produced the largest force ;
Shiffman (1992)	40	24-87	M: 20; F: 20	Strength, milk pouring, removing money from a wallet	Different prehension patterns and frequency, performance time ↑, hand strength ↓
Smith et al. (1999)	Y : 56 O : 38	20-58 66-87	M: 22; F: 34 M: 12; F: 26	Fine and coarse hand functions	Coarse motor time ↑, fine motor time ↑↑,
Frederiksen et al. (2006)	8342	45-98	n.a.	Measurement of hand grip strength during a follow-up of 4 years, using a hand dynamometer	Men showed more strength than women; hand grip strength showed an age effect.

Authors	N	Age (years)	Gender	Measurements	Main findings
Rahman et al. (2002)	O: 51	60-84	M: 9; F: 42	Assessment of grip and pinch strength by opening containers that were connected to a Jamar dynamometer through sensors	Grip and pinch strength were weakly related to the force needed to open most of the containers.
Mergl et al. (1959)	57	45 (± 20)	M: 25; F: 32	Drawing and writing tasks	Peak velocity ↓, speed ↓, movement automation ↓, writing pressure ↓
Morgan et al. (1994)	Y : 12 / O : 12	18-27 (21, 2) / 63-74 (69.9)	M: 6; F: 6 / M: 6; F: 6	Connecting targets with a zigzag pattern	Stroke duration ↑, pauses ↑, accuracy + peak velocity ↓

Table 1. Clinical studies examining the influence of aging on hand function. SMC: primary sensorimotor cortex; SMA: supplementary motor area; PMC: lateral premotor cortex; Y: young; O: old; 1*: first measurement; 2* second measurement; n.a.: no: available. M: male; F: female.

right hand was shorter when it was made towards the body (adductive movement) than away from the body (abductive movement) (Morgan et al., 1994). This finding refutes the theory that familiarity generates a positive effect, as the normal direction of the right hand during writing is away from the body (Morgan et al., 1994).

All in all, most of the evidence points to a decline in fine, complex, and gross hand motor function in older people, particularly after a certain age. Familiarity with the task does not always have a beneficial effect on performance.

5.2.2 Compensation

Although elderly subjects (50 years of age and older), compared to younger subjects, demonstrate a lower speed in hand motor activity, an increased activation in the contralateral sensorimotor cortex, lateral premotor area, supplementary motor area, and ipsilateral cerebellum has been observed (Mattay et al., 2002). Moreover, the elderly subjects showed activity in areas which were not active in younger subjects, i.e., ipsilateral sensorimotor cortex, putamen, and contralateral cerebellum (see table 2).

	Old	Young
Contralateral sensorimotor cortex	++	+
Lateral premotor cortex	++	+
Supplementary motor area	++	+
Ipsilateral cerebellum	++	+
Ipsilateral sensorimotor cortex	+	
Putamen	+	
Contralateral cerebellum	+	

Table 2. Activation of brain areas of older and younger people during hand motor activity. ++: more activity in the brain areas of old people, compared to the activity (+) in the brain areas of young people.

The increased activity in the aforementioned areas may reflect compensatory mechanisms (Mattay et al., 2002). In other words, motor activity of the hand of elderly subjects provokes a higher activity in areas which are also active in younger subjects and, in addition, activity in areas that are not active in younger persons (Mattay et al., 2002). Similar findings have been observed in a study in which older (mean age: 68 years) and younger (mean age: 26 years) subjects were asked to perform simple repetitive wrist and finger movements with the dominant hand (Hutchinson et al., 2002). Irrespective of the motor task (wrist or fingers), the older subjects in comparison with the younger subjects showed increased activity in the caudal supplementary motor area and ipsilateral supplementary motor cortex whereas contralateral primary sensorimotor cortex, premotor cortex, and supplementary motor cortex showed increased activation in the younger subjects. However, with respect to finger movements of both hands, the older subjects showed significantly more activity in the contralateral supplementary motor cortex (see table 3).

| | Dominant hand | |
	Old	Young
Caudal supplementary motor area	++	+
Ipsilateral supplementary motor area	++	+
Contralateral primary sensorimotor cortex	+	++
Contralateral premotor cortex	+	++
Contralateral supplementary motor cortex	+	++
	Both hands	
Contralateral supplementary motor cortex	++	+

Table 3. Increased (++) or normal (+) activity in brain areas of old and young people during the simple hand movement, performed by the dominant hand or by both hands

An explanation is that when the motor task becomes increasingly difficult as is the case in finger movements of the non-dominant hand, also older people are able to increase the activity in the contralateral supplementary motor cortex (Hutchinson et al., 2002). In other words, the higher the task demand, the more the motor network will be involved (Hutchinson et al., 2002).

In sum, to perform motor activity of the hand, older people are able to enhance and initiate activity in brain areas that are normally activated or not activated in younger people, respectively. The older person shows this pattern of activation to compensate for a decreased activation in areas that are normally or not activated in young people who perform the same hand motor activity.

5.3 Mild Cognitive Impairment and Alzheimer's Disease

Assessment results of fine hand motor function by applying the Finger-to-Thumb test (Franssen, Souren, Torossian, & Reisberg, 1999), Purdue Pegboard (Aggarwal, Wilson, Beck, Bienias, & Bennett, 2006), and a pointing/touching task (Camarda et al., 2007) revealed significant differences between older persons without dementia, older persons with Mild Cognitive Impairment, and Alzheimer patients. In these studies, Alzheimer patients performed worse than Mild Cognitive Impairment patients who, in turn, performed worse than the healthy controls (see table 4 for details on the diagnosis of Mild Cognitive Impairment and stage of Alzheimer's disease). However, when controlling for the presence of stroke, the Mild Cognitive Impairment patients did not perform significantly worse on the Purdue Pegboard than subjects with no cognitive impairments (Aggarwal et al., 2006).

Differences in the performance of the three groups were observed not only for fine hand motor activity but also for complex hand motor functions, which were assessed by the Assembly test of Purdue Pegboard, alternating movements of both hands, and Luria's three different movements by one hand (Kluger et al., 1997; Economou, Papageorgiou, Karageorgiou, & Vassilopoulos, 2007). In addition, patients with mild Alzheimer's disease performed slower on a task for gross hand motor function – finger tapping – than older persons without dementia (Kluger et al., 1997); a slower performance of finger tapping has not been confirmed in another study (Goldman, Baty, Buckles, Sahrmann, & Morris, 1999).

The discovery that gross hand motor activity, such as speed, is particularly affected in Alzheimer's disease has been confirmed at a somewhat more subtle level in studies using kinematic analyses of hand movements (table 4). These studies indicated that, compared with healthy controls, AD patients take longer to prepare movements, perform slower, show changing velocity profiles, and need more time to reach peak velocity. This latter symptom could be observed as a problem when initiating movements. In addition, they demonstrated variability in force when writing and when performing tasks in which a non-ink pen or a cursor had to be moved towards a target (Bellgrove et al., 1997; Ghilardi et al., 1999). Alzheimer patients showed more variation in velocity during writing not only in comparison with healthy controls, but with Mild Cognitive Impairment patients as well (Schröter et al., 2003). In contrast with healthy controls, Alzheimer patients showed signs of perseveration by writing more letters than required (Slavin, Phillips, Bradshaw, Hall, & Presnell, 1999). Furthermore, the handwriting of Alzheimer patients, and to a lesser extent of Mild Cognitive Impairment patients, was less automated and smooth than that of healthy controls (Schröter et al., 2003), thereby implying that a decline in hand movement coordination and automation, i.e., in fine hand motor activity, coincides with a decline in cognitive functioning (Schröter et al., 2003).

Taken together, Mild Cognitive Impairment patients and, to a larger extent, Alzheimer patients show impairment in fine and complex hand motor activity when compared with healthy older persons. Secondly, when compared with both healthy controls and Mild Cognitive Impairment patients, Alzheimer patients show impairment in gross motor activity, which is reflected primarily in a slower performance of hand motor function. Last but not least, Alzheimer patients may show signs of perseveration during writing tasks.

5.3.1 How the assessment of the hand motor function may support the diagnosis of (preclinical) dementia

The reviewed studies suggest that a relationship exists between hand motor function and cognitive status, similar to the one observed between gait and cognitive functioning (Scherder et al., 2007). For example, a decline in fine and complex hand motor function was observed to a much greater extent in Mild Cognitive Impairment patients than in older people with no cognitive impairment. However, the difference in fine hand motor function might disappear if Mild Cognitive Impairment patients with a stroke were excluded from data analysis (Aggarwal et al., 2006). It also emerged that older people and Mild Cognitive Impairment patients did not differ significantly in impairment of gross hand motor function. The assessment of hand motor function can differentiate more reliably between Alzheimer's disease and normal aging and between Alzheimer's disease and Mild Cognitive Impairment. Alzheimer patients showed the strongest impairment of fine, complex and gross hand motor function compared with healthy controls (Bellgrove et al., 1997; Ghilardi et al., 1999) and the patients with very mild AD (Goldman et al., 1999). To the best of my knowledge, only one study compared the hand motor function in vascular dementia patients with that of Mild Cognitive Impairment patients, Alzheimer patients, and older persons without dementia (Hall & Harvey, 2008). The results show that simple hand motor function, i.e., copying alternating hand-tapping performed by the examiner did not differentiate between the groups. The fact that this task did not involve alternating hand movements with a visuospatial component, strength, or speed might explain the absence of significant differences between the groups. All things considered, no firm conclusions can as yet be drawn about the (in)effectiveness of hand motor function as a tool to differentiate between the various subtypes of (preclinical) dementia.

The clinical outcome described above parallels the neuropathology characteristic of aging, Mild Cognitive Impairment and Alzheimer's disease. Activity in the frontoparietal network has been observed during a precision grip task and a sequence fist-edge-palm motor task (Ehrsson, Fagergren, & Forssberg, 2001; Umetsu et al., 2002). Frontoparietal connectivity is vulnerable in normal aging (Grieve, Williams, Paul, Clark, & Gordon, 2007), Mild Cognitive Impairment (Babiloni et al., 2007) and early Alzheimer's disease (Imran et al., 1999).

Authors	Age (years)	N	Stage	Gender	Measurement(s)	Main findings
Aggarwal et al. 2006	HC: 74.6 (6.7) MCI: 78.7 (7.0) AD: 81.9 (6.7)	558 198 60	n.a. n.a.	M:188, F: 370 M: 65, F: 133 M: 23, F: 37	Purdue Pegboard	AD versus MCI: Score Purdue Pegboard ↓ MCI versus HC: Score Purdue Pegboard ↓
Bellgrove et al. (1997)	HC: 73-88 AD: 73-88	12 12	MMSE 15-27	M:2; F:10 M:2; F:10	Connecting illuminated targets	Movement speed ↓, kinematic irregularities ↑, cycles of acceleration and deceleration ↑, time to prepare movements ↑, movement efficiency ↓, errors ↑
Camarda et al. 2007	HC: 69.7 (9.1) MCI: 69.7 (7.9) AD: 70.8 (6.4)	11 11 11	CDR 0.5 MMSE 17-24	M:5; F:6 M:5; F:6 M:5; F:6	Pointing at/touching illuminated targets	AD versus MCI/HC: ↓ reaction time, ↓ peak of acceleration, ↓ peak of velocity, ↓ peak of deceleration
Economou et al. 2007	HC: 58-88 (8.9) MCI: 62-90 (6.2) AD: 60-87 (8.2)	27 31 15	CDR 0.5 CDR 1.0	Unknown	Luria's alternating hand movements Luria's unimanual 3-stage movements	MCI versus HC: ↑ impairment on alternating movement test, ↓ uni-manual 3-stage movements AD versus MCI: ↑ impairment on alternating movement test, ↓ uni-man. 3-stage movements
Franssen et al. 1999	MCI: 72.6 (9.4) AD: 73.3 (7.70)	69 101	GDS 3 GDS 4	Unknown Unknown	Finger to thumb	MCI showed worse performance compared with cognitively intact people; AD patients performed worse than cognitively intact people
Ghilardi et al. (1999)	HC: 61-74 AD : 61-74	9 9		M:3; F:6 M:3; F:6	Moving a cursor to a target	Multiple curves in patient trajectories, discontinuous segments, changing velocity profiles
Goldman et al. 1999	HC: 73.2 (7.7) MCI: 72.0 (7.5) AD: 73.7 (7.8)	43 40 20	MMSE 9-24 CDR: 0 CDR 0.5 CDR 1	M: 21, F: 22 M: 19, F: 21 M: 9, F: 11	Finger tapping Reaction time and movement time on the Fitts task: movement of a stylus to a target	No differences on finger tapping between the three groups AD versus MCI: ↓ reaction time, ↓ movement time MCI versus HC: no differences
Hall & Harvey, 2008	HC MCI AD VaD Total group: 79.3 (65-94)	11 46 129 74	n.a. n.a. n.a. n.a.	Total group: M: 82, F:178	Finger tapping	No differences between groups
Kluger et al. (1997)	HC: 69.9 (8.6) MCI: 73.9 (8.2) AD: 71.6 (8.1)	41 25 25	GDS 3 GDS 4	M: 56.1% M: 56% M: 40%	Gross motor function: Finger-tapping speed, hand strength Fine motor function: Purdue & Grooved pegboard (dominant and non-dominant hand) Complex motor function: assembly test of Purdue Pegboard	MCI versus HC: Score Purdue Pegboard ↓, score Grooved Pegboard ↑, score assembly test Perdue Pegboard ↓ AD versus HC: Finger-tapping speed ↓, score Purdue Pegboard ↓, score Grooved Pegboard ↑, score assembly test of Perdue Pegboard ↓

Authors	Age (years)	N	Stage	Gender	Measurement(s)	Main findings
Schröter et al. (2003)	HC: 65.6 (7.9) MCI: 66.6 (11.1) AD : 70.6 (11.2)	40 39 35	MMSE 23-30 MMSE 15-30	M: 17; F:23 M: 16; F:23 M: 18; F:17	Task 1: drawing circles. Task 2: drawing circles while performing a second task	HC versus MCI: Number of changes of direction of velocity ↑ AD versus HC: Frequency of handwriting per day ↓, velocity variation ↑, relative velocity ↑, number of changes of direction of velocity ↑
Slavin et al. (1999)	HC: 66-88 AD: 66-88	16 16	MMSE 0-27	M:4; F:12 M:4; F:12	Writing four cursive l's in a single smooth movement at a comfortable speed	Stroke length variability ↑, stroke duration variability ↑, peak velocity variability ↑

Table 4: Studies examining the influence of Mild Cognitive Impairment (MCI), Alzheimer's Disease (AD) and vascular dementia (VaD) on hand function. n.a.: not available. CDR: Clinical Dementia Rating Scale [40]; GDS: Global Deterioration Scale [41]. M: male; F: female. HC: healthy controls.

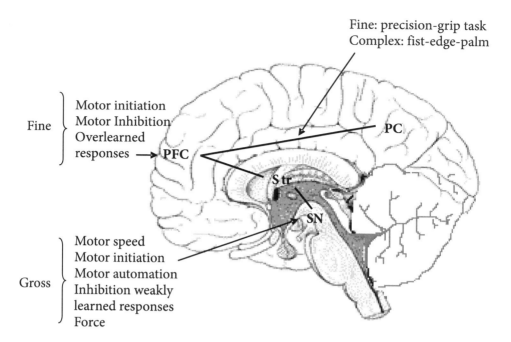

Figure 1. *The contribution of the frontostriatal, nigrostriatal and frontoparietal system to fine and gross motor-hand function. PFC: prefrontal cortex; Str: striatum; SN: substantia nigra; PC: parietal cortex. Fine: fine hand motor function; Gross: gross hand motor function.*

A dysfunction of the frontostriatal network due to a decline in the dopaminergic striatal innervation might cause impairment in gross hand motor function, such as motor speed (Sawamoto et al., 2007) (see figure 1). It should be stressed with respect to the present findings that, compared with normal aging, the striatum is more affected in Alzheimer patients, even in an early stage (Wolf et al., 1999).

5.3.2 Understanding higher level gait disturbances in mild dementia in order to improve rehabilitation; 'Last in - first out'

A phenomenon that could contribute to the understanding and prediction of disturbances in higher level gait and gait-related motor activity in the various subtypes of dementia is paraphrased as 'last in – first out'. 'Last in – first out' refers to the principle that neural circuits that mature late in development are the most vulnerable to neurodegeneration. The strength of relating symptoms to the 'last in – first out' principle is that a future symptom can be predicted and anticipated in a therapeutic way, even if the disease process has already started (see Chapter 6).

The 'last in – first out' principle will be addressed with respect to five neural networks: the superior longitudinal fasciculus, the uncinate fasciculus, the frontocerebellar and frontostriatal connections, and the cingulum.

'Last in – first out'

Gait disorders can be classified at three levels: lower level (musculoskeletal or peripheral nervous system disturbances), middle level (disturbances in e.g., basal ganglia, cerebellum) and higher level (disturbances in corticocortical and corticosubcortical connections, e.g., frontal connections with parietal lobes and frontal lobes with basal ganglia, respectively) (Thompson & Nutt, 2007). This chapter focuses on higher level gait disturbances.

Functional disturbances of higher level gait in an early stage of dementia have been understudied, in spite of the fact that disturbances in higher level gait and gait-related motor activity already occur in early stages of Alzheimer's disease, frontotemporal dementia (FTD), and vascular dementia (Scherder et al., 2007). Awareness of higher level gait disturbances in an early stage of dementia is clinically relevant as it has recently become clear that higher level gait is closely related to higher level cognitive functioning (Hausdorff, Yogev, Springer, Simon, & Giladi, 2005) such as executive functions, e.g., attention and planning (Mulder & Hochstenbach, 2003). Epidemiological studies support a close relationship between higher level gait and cognitive functioning (Rosano et al., 2005; Verghese, Wang, Lipton, Holtzer, & Xue, 2007). It has been suggested that participating in a physically active lifestyle may protect against dementia (Fratiglioni et al., 2004; Rovio et al., 2005). Similarly, a disturbance in higher level gait and gait-related motor activity that causes a decrease in the level of physical activity, such as walking, coincides with a decline in cognitive functioning (Rosano et al., 2005). In addition, a decrease in the level of physical activity, for example, slowing gait, might even predict dementia (Waite et al., 2005).

The close relationship between higher level gait and cognitive functioning makes it clinically relevant to understand and predict which aspects of higher level gait and gait-related motor activity will be either preserved or disturbed during the course of Alzheimer's disease, frontotemporal dementia, or vascular dementia. I suggest that a phenomenon known as 'retrogenesis' might contribute to the understanding and prediction of disturbances in higher level gait and gait-related motor activity in the various subtypes of dementia. Retrogenesis implies that the progression of degeneration follows the course of normal maturation in reverse order (Thompson et al., 2007; Reisberg et al., 2002). In other words, brain circuits that mature late in ontogenesis are most vulnerable to early neurodegeneration. This principle, paraphrased as 'last in – first out', also implies the opposite: neuronal circuits that mature early are less vulnerable to early neurodegeneration. Retrogenesis has been described in Alzheimer's disease for functional abilities, cognition, emotion, neurologic release signs, biomolecular markers, and neuropathology (Braak & Braak, 1996; Reisberg et al., 2002). Aspects of retrogenesis may also be present in other subtypes of dementia such as frontotemporal dementia and vascular dementia (Reisberg et al., 2002). The clinical relevance of retrogenesis is that one can understand and predict the next cognitive and behavioural disturbances, allowing optimization of care (Reisberg et al., 2002). A major strength of the 'last in – first out' principle is, in addition, that it allows the understanding and prediction of which functions will be disturbed or preserved at an early stage of dementia; the stage in which therapeutic strategies are the most effective (Tedeschi, Cirillo, Tessitore, & Cirillo, 2008).

Prediction of disturbances in higher level gait and gait-related motor activity during the course of Alzheimer's disease, frontotemporal dementia, and vascular dementia, would enable one to anticipate an upcoming disability or further deterioration and train patients at a stage in which the disability is not yet present or not that severe, and thus hopefully postponing or attenuating the diminishment of function. This information can contribute to our understanding of disturbances in higher level gait and gait-related motor activity in dementia and can subsequently be incorporated into rehabilitation programmes, in order to test their potential effectiveness (see Chapter 6).

5.3.3 Outline

Firstly, I briefly present the brain regions that are structurally and functionally connected by the five neuronal networks, followed by the degeneration of the networks in mild dementia. Subsequently, the stage of structural maturation and degeneration of each network in three major subtypes of dementia: Alzheimer's disease, frontotemporal dementia, and vascular dementia, in the context of the 'last in – first out' hypothesis will be addressed.

Then I deal with the role that each network plays in higher level gait and briefly explain the pathological higher level gait pattern in a mild stage of each subtype of dementia. Following this, in the context of the 'last in – first out' hypothesis, some theoretical considerations about possible stage-related rehabilitation strategies for each subtype of dementia are presented in the next chapter.

Nomenclature

As Brodmann areas are seldom mentioned in studies and the relationship between Brodmann areas and specific brain regions varies in the literature, two researchers studied the literature independently and reached the following consensus: BA4: primary motor cortex; BA6,8: premotor and supplementary motor cortex/superior frontal cortex; BA9,46,10: dorsolateral prefrontal cortex (DLPFC)/middle frontal gyrus; BA44,45,47: ventrolateral prefrontal cortex (VLPFC)/inferior frontal gyrus; BA11,12: orbitofrontal cortex; BA32: anterior cingulate cortex (ACC); BA24,25: the subgenual ACC; BA29,30,31: posterior cingulate cortex (PCC); BA1,2,3: primary somatosensory areas; BA7: superior and inferior parietal cortex, intraparietal cortex, secondary somatosensory cortex; BA39: gyrus angularis; BA40: gyrus supramarginalis; BA39,40: also inferior parietal lobe; BA22: superior temporal gyrus; BA20: inferior/middle temporal gyrus; BA38: anterior temporal pole; BA28: entorhinal cortex/uncus; BA34,35: (para) hippocampal region, amygdala; BA18,19: visual association areas, cuneus/precuneus, lingual and fusiform gyrus.

Five neuronal networks and connected brain regions
related to higher level gait

↓

Structural degeneration of the five neuronal networks in mild dementia

↓

Structural maturation in relation to degeneration of the five neuronal circuits
in mild dementia ('last in – first out')

Contribution of the five neuronal networks to higher level gait disturbances
in mild dementia

Theoretical considerations about possible stage-related rehabilitation strategies for each subtype
of dementia

Diagram 1.

Five networks associated with higher level gait and gait-related motor activity

In this section the brain regions that are connected by the five neuronal networks will be described as well as the extent to which the five neuronal networks are affected in an early stage of dementia.

5.3.4 Superior longitudinal fasciculus (SLF)

Brain regions connected by the SLF

In humans, the superior longitudinal fasciculus (SLF) connects the frontal lobe with the parietal, temporal (Wernicke's area; superior temporal gyrus, temporal pole), and occipital lobes (visual association areas) (Bürgel et al., 2006; Catani, Howard, Pajevic, & Jones, 2002). More specifically, in the monkey brain, the primary, premotor, and supplementary motor cortex, the DLPFC and the VLPFC, are connected with the primary somatosensory cortex, the superior and inferior parietal cortex/secondary somatosensory cortex, and the inferior parietal lobe, that is, supramarginal gyrus and angular gyrus (Schmahmann et al., 2007) (figure 2).

Degeneration of SLF in mild dementia

In a mild and a mild to moderate stage of Alzheimer's disease, a decrease of the frontoparietal and frontotemporal resting-state functional connectivity has been observed (Stam et al., 2006; Wang et al., 2007). In the same population, compared to controls, fractional anisotropy (FA), which may reflect myelination and connectivity, was significantly reduced in the bilateral SLF (Parente et al. 2008; Rose et al., 2000). FA reduction in the SLF has also been observed in a mild stage of both frontal and temporal variants of frontotemporal dementia (fFTD and tFTD, respectively) (Borroni et al., 2007). The SLF has not been examined in vascular dementia.

'Last in – first out'

The SLF is one of the least developed tracts in newborns (0-12 months) (Hermoye et al., 2006). It develops slowly during the first five years of postnatal life (Zhang et al., 2007) and continues to develop into adulthood (Giorgio et al., 2008). The 'last in – first out' phenomenon holds only for early stage Alzheimer's disease and frontotemporal dementia. In other words, the SLF matures late and is affected in the early stages of Alzheimer's disease and frontotemporal dementia (table 5).

Contribution to gait and gait disturbances in mild dementia

SLF. We suggest that an early disturbance in the awareness of limb and trunk location in body-centred space, a gait-related function of the SLF (Schmahmann et al., 2007), may contribute to a decline in postural stability, to wide base and to involuntary trunk movements, characteristic of early gait disturbances in Alzheimer's disease, frontotemporal dementia, and vascular dementia (Scherder et al., 2007) (table 5). As table 5 shows, no-one has so far attempted to ascertain the extent of structural degeneration of the SLF in vascular dementia

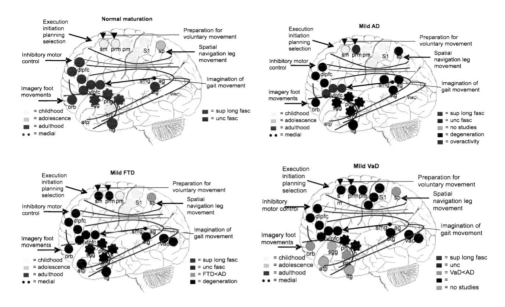

Figure 2. Some major gait-related functions of brain regions belonging to the superior longitudinal fasciculus (sup long fasc) and uncinate fasciculus (unc fasc) during normal structural maturation and in a mild stage of Alzheimer's disease (AD), frontotemporal dementia (FTD) and vascular dementia (VaD) (table 1). S1: primary somatosensory areas; sp: superior parietal cortex; pm: primary motor cortex; prm: premotor cortex; sm: supplementary motor cortex; dlpfc: dorsolateral prefrontal cortex; vlpfc: ventrolateral prefrontal cortex; sgg: subgenual gyrus; phg: parahippocampal gyrus; H: hippocampus; orb: orbitofrontal cortex; atp: anterior temporal pole; itg: inferior temporal gyrus; erc: entorhinal cortex; smg: supramarginal gyrus; ag: angular gyrus; stg: superior temporal gyrus; vac: visual association cortex.

Brain regions belonging to SLF. Gait-related functions of brain regions belonging to the SLF that are vulnerable in early Alzheimer's disease include action representation/motor imagery, motor inhibition, alternating foot movements and observational modelling on movement dynamics. Action representation/motor imagery and motor inhibition also show a decline in early stage frontotemporal dementia and vascular dementia (table 4). We suggest that a decline in motor imagery might contribute to a decline in postural stability and to wide-base walking, as observed in early stage Alzheimer's disease and vascular dementia (table 4). Indeed, the superior parietal lobe is one of the structures that is involved in motor imagery of postural control and precise foot placement during gait (Bakker et al., 2008).

5.3.5 Uncinate fasciculus

Brain regions connected by the uncinate fasciculus (UF)
In humans, connections exist between the orbitofrontal cortex, DLPFC, the sub-genual ACC, and the anterior and inferior lateral temporal lobe. Other connections exist between the former mentioned areas and the medial temporal region, that is, entorhinal cortex, amygdala (ventral part), and (para)hippocampal gyrus (Catani et al., 2002; Ebeling & von Cramon, 1992; Kier, Staib, Davis, & Bronen, 2004) (figure 2).

Degeneration of UF in mild dementia
In Alzheimer patients who were mildly to severely cognitively impaired, FA values were significantly reduced, compared to the control group (Taoka et al., 2006). Already in a preclinical stage of familial frontotemporal dementia, asymptomatic carriers of the progranulin mutation gene showed an FA reduction, indicating a decline in UF (Borroni et al., 2008). In vascular dementia, the UF itself has not been examined.

'Last in – first out'
Maturation of the UF has been observed until the age of at least 17 (Eluvathingal, Hasan, Kramer, Fletcher, & Ewing-Cobbs, 2007). As there is no information about the extent of the maturation of the UF network above the age of 17 and the UF itself has not been examined in vascular dementia, no firm conclusions can be drawn about the presence/absence of the 'last in – first out' phenomenon for this disorder. The 'last in – first out' phenomenon does, however, hold for the majority of the separate UF-related brain regions connected with Alzheimer's disease and frontotemporal dementia (table 6).

Contribution to gait and gait disturbances in mild dementia
UF. A disturbance in gait-related UF functions, such as imagery of foot movement sequences and naming human actions, may explain a decrease in stride length and walking velocity in early Alzheimer's disease and apractic gait in early vascular dementia (table 3). For example, imagery-based gait training has been shown to improve stride length and gait speed in stroke patients (Dunsky, Dickstein, Ariav, Deutsch, & Marcovitz, 2006). A deficit in naming motor actions coincided with a deficit in processing these same actions (object use) on verbal command, i.e., apraxia (Smith & Bryson, 2007).

Brain regions belonging to UF. Gait-related functions of brain regions belonging to the UF that are vulnerable in early Alzheimer's disease, frontotemporal dementia and vascular dementia and which do not overlap with the SLF (above) include spatial navigation and head and trunk stabilization (table 6). Impairment in these two functions, besides the SLF, might contribute to the decline in postural stability in early Alzheimer's disease (O'Keeffe et al., 1996) and vascular dementia (Morgan et al., 2007) and involuntary trunk movements in frontotemporal dementia (Mendez, Shapira, & Miller., 2005).

5.3.6 Frontocerebellar connections

Brain regions connected by frontocerebellar connections

The medial cerebellum is connected to the primary motor cortex (Schubotz & von Cramon, 2001), and the premotor and supplementary cortices (Ridler et al., 2006). The lateral region of the cerebellum, including the dentate nucleus, is functionally connected to the inferior frontal gyrus (pars opercularis and pars triangularis) and the DLPFC (Rao et al., 1997; Tamada, Miyauchi, Imamizu, Yoshioka, & Kawato, 1999) (figure 3).

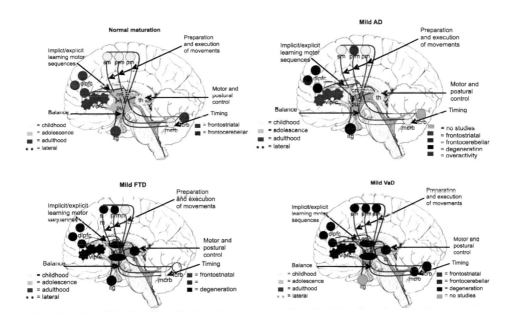

Figure 3. Some major gait-related functions of brain regions belonging to the frontostriatal and frontocerebellar connections during normal maturation, and in a mild stage of Alzheimer's disease (AD), frontotemporal dementia (FTD) and vascular dementia (VaD) (table 1). pm: primary motor cortex; prm: premotor cortex; sm: supplementary motor cortex; dlpfc: dorsolateral prefrontal cortex; vlpfc: ventrolateral prefrontal cortex; cn: caudate nucleus; pu: putamen; th: thalamus; mcrb: medial cerebellum; lcrb: lateral cerebellum.

Degeneration of frontocerebellar connections in mild dementia
Primary cortical areas and cerebellum are relatively preserved in mild Alzheimer's disease (Mielke & Heiss, 1998). In contrast, mild frontotemporal dementia patients showed a higher activation in the cerebellum during a working memory task than Alzheimer patients, probably to compensate for the decrease in frontal activation (Rombouts et al., 2003). Concerning vascular dementia, no studies are available.

'Last in – first out'
The connection between the premotor and supplementary motor cortex and medial cerebellum matures early whereas the connection between the middle and inferior frontal gyri and the posterolateral cerebellum matures late (Ridler et al., 2006).

Structural maturation and neuropathology have not been studied in relation to frontocerebellar connections as an entity. Within these limits, the present findings suggest that the 'last in – first out' phenomenon may hold for Alzheimer's disease, implying that the connection between the motor cortex and the (medial) cerebellum matures early and is not affected in the early stages of Alzheimer's disease (table 5).

Contribution to gait and gait disturbances in mild dementia
Frontocerebellar connections. By coordinating limb movements the frontocerebellar circuit may contribute to steadiness. Indeed, in patients with cerebellar degeneration, an impairment in lower extremity coordination does cause postural instability (Hudson & Krebs, 2000). This is a clinical symptom of early stage vascular dementia (Morgan et al., 2007). The relationship between upright posture and equilibrium is expressed in the observation that lack of attention to restore upright stance increases the risk of impaired balance (Brown, Shumway-Cook, & Woollacott, 1999). Disequilibrium is part of early gait disturbances in Alzheimer's disease (Morgan et al., 2007).

Brain regions belonging to frontocerebellar connections. Apart from the cerebellum, brain regions belonging to the frontocerebellar connections show an overlap with the brain regions of the SLF. Consequently, we refer to the SLF for the contribution of an impairment in these gait-related functions to gait disturbances in early stage Alzheimer's disease, frontotemporal dementia and vascular dementia.

5.3.7 Frontostriatal connections

Brain regions connected by the frontostriatal connections
In the human brain, two bundles connect the primary motor cortex and the DLPFC with the lateral and medial putamen, whereas the premotor area is con-

nected with the dorsal posterior putamen (Leh, Ptito, Chakravarty, & Strafella, 2007). The supplementary motor area and the VLPFC are connected with the ventral anterior caudate nucleus; the DLPFC shows a functional relationship with the dorsal posterior caudate nucleus (Leh et al., 2007).The caudate nucleus and putamen project to the thalamus and cerebellum (both areas not further specified) (Leh et al., 2007) (figure 3).

Degeneration of frontostriatal connections in mild dementia

In humans, frontostriatal degeneration is not characteristic for Alzheimer's disease (Rabinovici et al., 2007). Mild to moderate frontotemporal dementia patients (fFTD, semantic dementia, progressive nonfluent aphasia: PNA) show more atrophy in the frontostriatal network than Alzheimer patients (Rabinovici et al., 2007). Frontostriatal connections have not been examined in vascular dementia.

'Last in – first out'

The maturation of the frontostriatal connections has been observed during the transition from childhood to mid-adulthood (table 5) (Rubia et al., 2006). The 'last in – first out' phenomenon holds only for the frontostriatal network in frontotemporal dementia. Furthermore, it does not hold for the majority of the separate brain regions related to the fronto-striatal connections, irrespective of the subtype of dementia (table 6).

Contribution to gait and gait disturbances in mild dementia

Frontostriatal connections. Obviously, an impairment in self-initiated automatic movements (Bartels & Leenders, 2008) and movement initiation (Herrero, Barcia, & Navarro, 2002) will lead to a deficit in initiating motor activity in early stage frontotemporal dementia (de Mendonça, Ribeiro, Guerreiro, & Garcia, 2004). In addition, freezing gait, characteristic of early stage vascular dementia, is triggered by a disturbance in gait initiation (Snijders et al., 2008).

Brain regions belonging to the frontostriatal connections. The frontal areas belonging to the frontostriatal connections overlap with the SLF; hence we refer to the SLF for an overview of the contribution of an impairment in these gait-related functions to gait disturbances in early stage Alzheimer's disease, frontotemporal dementia and vascular dementia. The caudate nucleus and putamen, as well as the thalamus, and their gait-related functions (implicit visuomotor sequence learning and balance control) degenerate in early stage frontotemporal dementia and vascular dementia (table 6). An impairment in balance control may contribute to a decline in postural stability (Rival, Ceyte, & Olivier, 2005) as observed in early vascular dementia and to a deficit in initiating motor activity, characteristic of early frontotemporal dementia. It should be noted with a view to the relationship between balance and motor initiation that functional balance training improved gait initiation in older persons (de Bruin, Swanenburg, Betschon, & Murer, 2009).

5.3.8 Cingulum

Brain regions connected by the cingulum

The longest cingular pathway connects the uncus and parahippocampal gyrus to the subrostral areas of the frontal lobe (orbitofrontal cortex) (Bürgel et al., 2006; Catani et al., 2002). Short pathways of the cingulum connect the medial frontal gyrus, posterior parietal lobe, cuneus, lingual, and fusiform gyrus (visual association areas) with each other (Catani et al., 2002). In rhesus monkeys, the supplementary motor cortex, the DLPFC, the orbitofrontal cortex, and the (subgenual) ACC are connected with the inferior parietal lobe and the retrosplenial cortex (Morris, Petrides, & Pandya, 1999; Schmahmann et al., 2007) (figure 4).

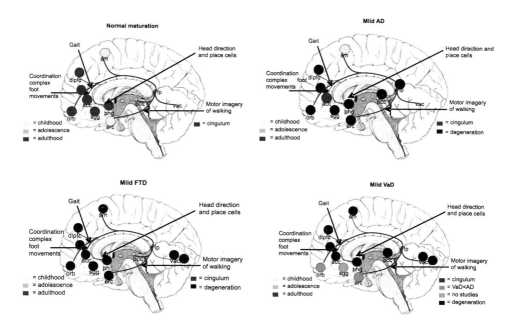

Figure 4. Some major gait-related functions of brain regions belonging to the cingulum during normal maturation, and in a mild stage of Alzheimer's disease (AD), frontotemporal dementia (FTD) and vascular dementia (VaD) (table 3). sm: supplementary motor cortex; dlpfc: dorsolateral prefrontal cortex; acc: anterior cingulate cortex; orb: orbitofrontal cortex; sgg: subgenual anterior cingulate; phg: parahippocampal gyrus; erc: entorhinal cortex; pcc: posterior cingulate cortex (retrosplenial cortex); ip: inferior parietal lobe; vac: visual association cortex.

Degeneration of the cingulum in mild dementia

FA was not reduced in the entire cingulum in mild Alzheimer patients, compared to controls (Naggara et al., 2006). At a more specific level, however, a decrease in FA is particularly characteristic for the PCC in mild to moderate Alzheimer patients (Parente et al., 2008) whereas the ACC is relatively preserved (Frisoni et al., 2007). Furthermore, irrespective of the subtype of frontotemporal dementia (tau, ubiqutin, fFTD, tFTD, PNA), cingulate atrophy was observed in a mild stage showed, compared to controls (Barnes et al., 2007). Atrophy was observed more anterior in mild frontotemporal dementia (ACC) and more posterior in Alzheimer's disease (Barnes et al., 2007; Borroni et al., 2007; Richards et al., 2009). Patients with ischemic stroke and mild vascular cognitive decline show atrophy in the ACC, central gyrus, and PCC (Stebbins et al., 2008; Grau-Olivares et al., 2007). The ACC is also affected in mild to moderate SIVD (Shim et al., 2006; Yang et al., 2002). Of note is that the hypometabolism in the ACC in mild vascular dementia patients is more severe than in Alzheimer's disease (Kerrouche, Herholz, Mielke, Holthoff, & Baron, 2006).

'Last in – first out'

The cingulum and its separate parts such as the ACC, subgenual ACC and the PCC, continue to mature into adulthood (Eshel, Nelson, Blair, Pine, & Ernst., 2007; Marsh et al., 2006; Rubia, Smith, Taylor, & Brammer, 2007). With respect to the cingulum as an entity, the 'last in – first out' phenomenon applies to fronto-temporal dementia and vascular dementia (table 5). Furthermore, despite its late maturation, the cingulum itself is not affected in mild Alzheimer's disease (table 5). This is in stark contrast with a number of separate brain regions to which it is connected, such as the entorhinal cortex, the (para) hippocampal region, the inferior parietal lobe and the PCC (table 6).

Stage of structural degeneration and gait disturbances in dementia

Five neuronal circuits	Contribution of five neuronal circuits to gait	Stage of structural maturation	AD		FTD		VaD	
			Stage of struct. degen.	Early gait disturbances	Stage of struct. degen.	Early gait disturbances	Stage of struct. degen.	Early gait disturbances
SLF	Awareness of limb and trunk location in body-centred space[1,†]	adulthood[2]	early[3]	Decrease in postural stability[4] Wide base[5]	early[6]	Involuntary trunk movements[7]	ns	Decrease in postural stability[8] Wide base[9]
UF	Imaging of sequences of foot movements[10]	adolescence[11]	early[12]	Decrease in steplength[13] and walking velocity[13]	early[6]		ns	Small step gait[14] Slow stepping[8] Apractic/ataxic gait[15]
Fronto-cerebellar connections	Coordination of limb movements[16] Upright posture[18*]	childhood (Front/mot-med. crbl.)[17] adulthood (Inf front-lat. crbl.)[17]	ns ns	Dis-equilibrium[4]	ns ns		ns ns	Unsteadiness[8]
Frontostriatal connections	Spatial information necessary for gait[19] Movement initiation, planning[23]	adulthood[20]	late[21]		early[21]	Deficit in initiating motor activity[22]	ns	Start hesitation or freezing[9] Freezing upon turning[9]

Stage of structural degeneration and gait disturbances in dementia

Five neuronal circuits	Contribution of five neuronal circuits to gait	Stage of structural maturation	AD		FTD		VaD	
			Stage of struct. degen.	Early gait disturbances	Stage of struct. degen.	Early gait disturbances	Stage of struct. degen.	Early gait disturbances
Cingulum	Coordination, maintenance, and retrieval of complex foot movement sequences[24-25]	adulthood[26]	late[27]		early[28]		early[29]	Unsteadiness[8] Apractic[15]

Table 5. Table 5 shows the role of five neuronal circuits in higher level gait and gait disturbances in early stage Alzheimer's disease (AD), vascular dementia (VaD), and frontotemporal dementia (FTD). The table also demonstrates in which subtype of dementia neuronal circuits mature late (adolescence/adulthood) and degenerate early (childhood) and vice versa ('last in – first out' phenomenon) The structural maturation stage and the stages of structural degeneration in the three subtypes of dementia that follow the 'last in – first out' phenomenon are highlighted yellow in the table. SLF: superior longitudinal fasciculus; UF: Uncinate fasciculus. Front/mot-med. crbl: primary, premotor, and supplementary cortices of the frontal lobe connected to the medial cerebellum; Inf front-lat. crbl.: inferior frontal gyrus and dorsolateral prefrontal cortex connected to the lateral cerebellum; ns=not studied; Stage of struct. degen.: stage of structural degeneration; *This function was not related to gait in the referred study; ⁺study concerned monkeys.

[1]Schmahmann et al., 2007; [2]Giorgio et al., 2008; [3]Parente et al., 2008; [4]Nakamura et al., 1997; [5]O'Keeffe et al., 1996; [6]Borroni et al., 2007; [7]Mendez et al., 2005; [8]Pugh and Lipsitz, 2002; [9]Verghese et al., 2007a; [10]Jackson, Lafleur, Malouin, Richards, & Doyon, 2003; [11]Eluvathingal et al., 2007; [12]Taoka et al., 2006; [13]Goldman et al., 1999; [14]Tanaka et al., 1995; [15]Poljasvaara et al., 2003; [16]Debaere et al., 2001; [17]Ridler et al., 2006; [18]Ouchi et al., 2004; [19]Bartels and Leerders, 2008; [20]Rubia et al., 2006; [21]Rabinovici et al., 2007; [22]de Mendonça et al., 2004; [23]Herrero et al., 2002; [24]Lafleur et al., 2002; [25]Heuninckx, Wenderoth, Debaere, Peeters, & Swinnen, 2005; [26]Dubois et al., 2006; [27]Naggara et al., 2006; [28]Barnes et al., 2007; [29]Stebbins et al., 2008.

Gait-related motor functions of brain regions belonging to the five neuronal circuits		Functional maturation-stage of gait-related motor functions			Stage of structural degeneration		
Frontal lobe	Gait-related motor functions*	Gait-related motor functions with maturation stage	Functional maturation stage	Structural maturation stage	AD	FTD	VaD
Primary motor cortex	Preparation and execution of movements[1]	Execution of walking[2]	childhood	childhood[3]	late[4]	late[5]	early[6]
Premotor/supplementary motor cortex	Execution, learning, initiation, planning, sequence, selection, and observation of movements[7,8,9]	Effect of observational modelling on movement[10]; Planning of movements[11,12]	childhood childhood	childhood[3]	late[13]	early[14]	early[15]
Dorsolateral prefrontal cortex	Inhibitory motor control, motor imagery[16,17]	Action representation system/motor imagery[18] Motor inhibition[21]	adulthood adolescence	adulthood[19]	early[20]	early[14]	early[15]
Ventrolateral prefrontal cortex	Imagery of foot movements[7]	Motor imagery[18]	adulthood	adulthood[22]	late[23]	early[24]	early[25]
Orbitofrontal cortex	Sequence of foot movements by motor imagery[26]	Motor imagery[18]	adulthood	adulthood[19]	early[27]	early[28]	early[6]
Parietal lobe							
Primary somatosensory areas	Sensori-motor integration[29]	Sensori-motor integration[30]	childhood	childhood[3]	late[4]	late[31]	early[15]
Superior parietal lobe	Imagination of standing and walking; imagination of precision gait; spatial navigation of leg movement[32,33]	Action representation system/motor imagery[18]	adolescence	adolescence[3]	early[34]	early[34]	early[6]
Inferior parietal lobe	Executing sequential foot movements[35]	Decrease associated movements with age for alternating foot movements[36]	adolescence	adolescence/adulthood[37]	early[38]	mid[39]	mid[40]
	Observation and imagery of gait movement[41]	Observational modelling on movement dynamics[37]	adulthood				
Superior temporal gyrus	Imagery and observation of standing, walking and running[42,43]	Action representation system/motor imagery[18]	adolescence	adulthood[3]	early[44]	early[14]	early[45]
Entorhinal cortex; (para) hippocampal region	Spatial planning; navigation/ imagination of the environment[41,46,47]; Head direction and place cells/spatial navigation[51]	Spatial navigation[48]	adulthood	childhood[3]	early[49]	early[50]	early[39]
		Head- and trunk stabilization under normal vision[52]	adulthood	adulthood[53]	early[54]	early[14]	early[45]

Occipital lobe

Visual association areas[55]	Visual input during bipedal locomotor activities[55]					
	Less dependent on visual information during maturation[56]	adulthood	ns	late[57]	early[58]	early[40]
Striatum						
Caudate nucleus/putamen	Execution of well-learned sequences[45-59], explicit and implicit learning of motor Sequences[60,59,62,63]; Balance[64]	adulthood	adolescence[61]	mid[66]	early[67]	early[15,68]
	Implicit visuomotor sequence learning[60]					
	Balance control[65]	adulthood	adolescence[61]	mid[66]	early[67]	
Thalamus	Motor and postural control[69]	childhood	childhood[71]	late[72]	early[5]	early[73]
	Static standing balance[70]					
Cingulum						
Anterior cingulate cortex	Gait[74], Coordination complex foot movements[75]	adolescence	adulthood[22]	late[77]	early[78]	early[45]
	Stride-to-stride control of walking[76]					
Posterior cingulate cortex	Motor imagery of walking[?]	adolescence	adolescence[79]	early[80]	mid[78]	early[15]
	Action representation system/motor imagery[30]					
Cerebellum	Timing and motor coordination lower extremities, including foot placement[81,83]	ns[a]	childhood[MCRB85] adulthood[LCRB85]	ns[a]	ns[a]	ns[a]
	Lower limb coordination[84]					

Table 6. Main gait-related motor functions of the *separate* brain areas belonging to the superior longitudinal fasciculus, uncinate fasciculus, frontostriatal connections, fronto-cerebellar connections and cingulum, and stage of maturation. *Information extracted from animal experimental and human studies (healthy subjects and patients, irrespective of age). ns: not studied. ns[a]: concerning the functional maturation stage of gait-related motor functions and stage of structural degeneration, a distinction between medial and lateral cerebellum has not been made in literature. MCRB: medial cerebellum; LCRB: lateral cerebellum.

[1]Suzuki, Miyai, Ono, & Kubota; [2]Roncesvalles et al., 2000; [3]Gogtay et al., 2004; [4]Braak and Braak, 1991; [5]Diehl-Schmid et al., 2007; [6]Kerrouche et al., 2006; [7]Binkofski and Buccino, 2006; [8]Cunnington, Windischberger, & Moser, 2005; [9]Rushworth, Walton, Kennerley, & Bannerman, 2004; [10]Ashford, Davids, & Bennett, 2007; [11]Claxton, Keen, & McCarty, 2003; [12]von Hofsten, 2004; [13]Ouchi et al., 2004; [14]Borroni et al., 2007; [15]Grau-Oliveres et al., 2007; [16]Kelly et al., 2004; [17]Malouin et al., 2003; [18]Choudbury, Charman, Bird, & Blakemore, 2007; [19]Segalowitz and Davies, 2004; [20]Kashani et al., 2008; [21]Rubia et al., 2000; [22]Eshel et al., 2007; [23]Halliday, Double, Macdonald, & Kril, 2003; [24]Ibach et al., 2004; [25]Kuczynski, Jagust, Chui, & Reed, 2009; [26]Jackson et al., 2003; [27]Frisoni, Prestia, Rasser, Bonetti, & Thompson, 2009; [28]Nyatsanza et al., 2003; [29]Christensen et al., 2007; [30]Metcalfe et al., 2005; [31]Rosén, Gustafson, & Risberg, 1993; [32]Oleser, Nagy, Westerberg, & Klingberg, 2003; [33]Bakker et al., 2008; [34]Varrone et al., 2002; [35]Lafleur et al., 2002; [36]Gasser, Rousson, Caflisch, & Largo, 2007; [37]Oleser, Nagy, Westerberg, & Klingberg, 2003; [38]Kobayashi et al., 2003; [39]Du et al., 2007;[40]Stebbins et al., 2008; [41]Iseki, Hanakawa, Shinozaki, Nankaku, & Fukuyama, 2008; [42]Barraclough, Xiao, Oram, & Perrett, 2006; [43]Jahn et al., 2004; [44]Lüth et al., 2005; [45]Shim, Yang, Kim, Shon, & Chung; [46]Sargolini et al., 2006; [47]Sheridan and Hausdorff, 2007; [48]Nardini, Jones, Fedford, & Braddick, 2008; [49]Hirao et al., 2006; [50]Richards et al., 2009; [51]Rolls, 1999; [52]Assaiante and Amblard, 1993; [53]Casey, Thomas, Davidson, Kunz, & Franzen, 2002; [54]Villain et al., 2008; [55]Fukuyama et al., 1997; [56]Vallis and McFadyen, 2005; [57]Meltzer et al., 1996; [58]Eslinger et al., 2007; [59]Jueptner et al., 1997; [60]Thomas et al., 2004; [61]Kirshenbaum, Riach, & Starkes, 2001; [62]Floyer-Lea and Matthews, 2004; [63]Roy, Phillips, & Beaulieu, 2005; [64]Rosano, Aizenstein, Studenski, & Newman, 2007; [65]Kirshenbaum, Riach, & Starkes, 2001; [66]Cousins et al., 2003; [67]Kim et al., 2007; [68]Yang et al., 2002; [69]García-Cabezas, Rico, Sánchez-González, & Cavada, 2007; [70]Rival et al., 2005; [71]Zhang et al., 2005; [72]Luckhaus et al., 2008; [73]Kato et al., 2008; [74]Hanakawa et al., 1999; [75]Heuninckx et al., 2005; [76]Scafetta et al., 2009; [77]Frisoni et al., 2007; [78]Barnes et al., 2007; [79]Marsh et al., 2006; [80]Parente et al., 2008; [81]D'Angelo and De Zeeuw, 2009; [82]Ivry, Keele, & Diener, 1988; [83]Stolze et al., 2002; [84]Cheron et al., 2001; [85]Ridler et al., 2006.

Contribution to gait and gait disturbances in mild dementia

Cingulum. Like the frontocerebellar connections, the cingulum is involved in co-ordination, maintenance and retrieval of complex foot movements (table 5). A disturbance in these functions may contribute to postural instability (Hudson & Krebs, 2000) in the early stages of vascular dementia.

Brain regions belonging to the cingulum. A number of brain regions belonging to the cingulum show an overlap with the SLF (supplementary motor cortex, DLPFC, inferior parietal lobe) and with the UF (orbitofrontal cortex). The anterior cingulate cortex and its role in stride-to-stride walking control (Scafetta, Marchi, & West, 2009) are affected in the early stages of frontotemporal dementia and vascular dementia. As stride-to-stride walking control is closely related to gait stability (Beauchet et al., 2009), an impairment may coincide with unsteadiness and a decline in postural stability as observed in the early stages of vascular dementia (table 5). The PCC shows degeneration in the early stages of Alzheimer's disease and vascular dementia. A disturbance in its function action representation system has been associated with limb apraxia (Leiguarda & Marsden, 2000) and might thus contribute to apractic gait in early vascular dementia (table 5).

Discussion

As presented in tables 5 and 6, the 'last in – first out' phenomenon or its opposite was not a fully consistent finding but differed for each subtype of dementia and type of network. One explanation for a lack of the 'last in – first out' phenomenon (e.g., entorhinal cortex) may be that in the majority of the studies reviewed here, the level of activity in a neuronal network or related brain region was considered to reflect the level of functional maturation. However, it has also been suggested that a higher neuronal activity in children compared to adults during the performance of a task would imply a compensation for being immature (Booth et al., 2003). This suggestion would weaken the presence of the 'last in – first out' phenomenon if the literature showed that a higher neuronal activity in a certain brain region in an early stage of maturation coincided with a late maturation of its related function. Therefore, we searched for studies that addressed exclusively the maturational stage of gait and gait-related motor functions. The combined data presented in table 6 show that the maturational stage of the different brain regions parallels the maturation stage of its main gait and gait-related motor functions.

There are other explanations for not finding the 'last in – first out' phenomenon in all cases (tables 5 and 6). For example, gender was not taken into consideration when discussing maturation of the five networks and related brain areas. Indeed, recent findings suggest that the rate of maturation of gray matter in, for example, the amygdala and hippocampus differs between boys and girls in close relationship to sex hormones (Neufang et al., 2009). However, in the majority of the maturation studies addressed in this review, gender was not mentioned or, only in very few studies, controlled for. Furthermore, age and gender are factors that should be taken into consideration when assessing variability in higher level gait. In people without dementia, stride time and step length show an age-related variability, due to loss of strength and flexibility (Kang & Dingwell, 2008). Similar age effects have been observed for standing and dynamic balance; in addition, women performed worse than men, indicating a more profound decline in postural control in women (Vereeck, Wuyts, Truijen, & van de Heyning, 2008). Furthermore, women appear to have weaker lower limb extensor strength than men (Musselman & Brouwer, 2005). As far as the authors know, lower limb functionalities have only been examined in Alzheimer's disease (Hebert, Scherr, McCann, Bienias, & Evans, 2008). In that study, a weaker lower limb extensor strength, together with a worse performance of a complete rotation task (360 degree turn) and an 8-foot walk task, have been observed in women compared to men. These and other variables (Morgan et al., 2007) should be taken into account in future assessments of higher level gait in dementia, in view of the paucity in studies in this area.

5.3.9 Physical activity; its relation with executive dysfunctions and depression

There are five separate but interconnected frontosubcortical systems (Pugh & Lipsitz, 2002). Precisely this close cooperation of the five systems explains why white matter lesions cause gait disturbance in combination with executive dysfunction (e.g., problem solving) and depression (Román, Erkinjuntti, Wallin, Pantoni, & Chui, 2002; Starr et al., 2003). Importantly, next to gait disturbances, executive dysfunction and depression may further reduce the level of physical activity, reflected in, among others, a decrease in (instrumental) activities of daily life (Kiosses & Alexopoulos, 2005; Wang et al., 2002). Therefore, the extent to which these latter two symptoms occur in the various subtypes of (preclinical) dementia is important to address.

Compared to elderly without cognitive impairment, patients with amnestic Mild Cognitive Impairment show a decline in executive functions but this decline remains within normal limits (van der Flier et al., 2002). Interestingly, among patients with Mild Cognitive Impairment, those who show a combination of memory deficits and executive dysfunctions are those who develop Alzheimer's disease (Guarch, Marcos, Salamero, & Blesa, 2004). Similarly, amnestic Mild Cognitive Impairment patients with depression have a two-fold increased risk for developing Alzheimer's disease, compared to those without depression (Modrego & Ferrández, 2004). The finding of this latter study implies that depression could be a clinical symptom of Mild Cognitive Impairment.

It has been observed in Alzheimer's disease that distraction further increased unsteadiness during walking, expressed in stride time variability (Sheridan, Solomont, Kowall, & Hausdorff, 2003). Distraction during walking implied that the patient read aloud a number of digits. Similar findings were observed in another study, in which Alzheimer patients showed a decrease in communication when walking was combined with talking (Cott, Dawson, Sidani, & Wells, 2002). To perform dual tasks, the patients have to divide attention, a cognitive function that heavily depends on executive functions. These findings suggest that also in Alzheimer's disease, executive dysfunction, expressed in an impaired performance in dual-tasks, has a close association with physical activities such as walking. Of the psychiatric disturbances, depression is the one that prevails the most in Alzheimer's disease (Lee & Lyketsos, 2003).

Results of a 5-year longitudinal study showed that the number of patients with vascular cognitive impairment no dementia (vCIND) who had problems with e.g., household activities and dressing, increased remarkably (Wentzel et al., 2001). Such a functional decline in both basic ADL and instrumental ADL (IADL) has been associated with psychomotor slowness (Nyenhuis et al., 2004), and with executive/attentional dysfunctions (Stephens et al., 2005). In another study with vascular cognitive impairment no dementia patients, a decline in functional capacity was expressed in a lower score on the Barthel Index (Frisoni, Galluzzi, Bresciani, Zanetti, & Geroldi., 2002). Furthermore, it has been observed that patients with vascular cognitive impairment no dementia are more depressed than elderly people without cognitive impairment (Nyenhuis et al., 2004).

In patients who could be classified as suffering from Subcortical ischaemic Vascular Dementia (SIVD; lacunar state and Binswanger's disease), a stepwise regression-analysis revealed that a decline in IADL, but not in basic ADL was significantly predicted by an impairment in executive/attentional functioning (Boyle, Cohen, Paul, Moser, & Gordon, 2002). This finding does not imply that basic ADL is not reduced in Subcortical ischaemic Vascular Dementia, as have been demonstrated recently (Pohjasvaara, Mantyla, Ylikoski, Kaste, & Erkinjuntti, 2003). In this latter study, patients with Subcortical ischaemic Vascular Dementia were more depressed than stroke patients without SIVD.

Patients with frontotemporal Mild Cognitive Impairment (FT-MCI) show executive dysfunctions among which attention deficits (de Mendonça et al., 2004). Depression has not been described in this group, as far as I know.

Finally, cognitive deficits in frontotemporal dementia are primarily characterized by executive dysfunctions (Perry & Hodges, 2000). In frontotemporal dementia the executive functions 'planning' and 'execution' of motor sequences was found to become progressively more difficult during the course of the disease (Talerico & Evans, 2001). Depression is not characteristic for frontotemporal dementia frontal variant but is a hallmark of the temporal variant (semantic dementia) (Bozeat, Gregory, Ralph, & Hodges, 2000).

Taken together, in all subtypes of (preclinical) dementia executive dysfunctions and depression are present, except for frontotemporal Mild Cognitive Impairment. Executive dysfunctions not only show a close association with a decline in physical activity, they may even predict it.

5.3.10 Physical activity; its relationship with energy expenditure and cognition

Already in normal aging, aerobic physical activity progressively declines, irrespective of whether older people are endurance-trained or sedentary (Wilson et al., 2000; Schilke, 1991). The reduction in aerobic physical activity in older persons is reflected in a decline in physical activity energy expenditure (Westerterp, 2000; Wilson & Morley, 2003). The rate of physical activity energy expenditure per day is often translated into metabolic equivalents (METs) (Weuve et al., 2004; Wang et al., 2004; Podewils et al., 2005). In one of the studies using METs, the level of physical energy expenditure of women without dementia was positively correlated with the level of cognitive functioning (Weuve et al., 2004). A biological basis for these findings emerges from a study with older persons without cognitive impairment which showed that the higher the level of aerobic fitness (expressed in Vo_2-max), the lower the age-related decline in tissue density in the frontal, parietal, and temporal lobe (Colcombe et al., 2003).

A more causal relationship has been demonstrated in a study in which healthy older people with an age ranging from 77-87 years participated (Evans et al., 2005). In that study, a high-intensity aerobic exercise program of 10-12 months enhanced cardiovascular fitness, reflected in an increase in aerobic power (Vo_2-max). Within this scope, the study of Kramer and co-workers (1999) is important since they showed that aerobic physical activity and not non-aerobic exercises, such as stretching, improved particularly executive functions in older people.

Of note is that women with cardiovascular risk factors such as hypertension and diabetes, showed the lowest level of expended energy. This is important since cardiovascular risk factors are also risk factors for Alzheimer's disease and even more for Subcortical ischaemic Vascular Dementia (Kivipelto et al., 2005; Román et al., 2002). In a recent prospective study, older people without dementia at baseline were followed during more than 5 years (Podewils et al., 2005). Similar to the previous study (Weuve et al., 2004), those with cardiovascular risk factors showed the lowest leisure-time energy expenditure (Podewils et al., 2005). In addition, they showed difficulties in more than one ADL and IADL (Podewils et al., 2005). They further observed a significant inverse relationship between leisure-time energy expenditure and the risk of Alzheimer's disease, i.e., the higher the leisure-time energy expenditure, the lower the risk of Alzheimer's disease. Of note is that a positive influence of increased physical activity, enhancing the level of energy-expenditure, on cognition has not been observed in patients with vascular dementia (Podewils et al., 2005). The authors indicate that also other studies (e.g., Yoshitake et al., 1995) failed to find a lowering effect of physical activity on the risk of vascular dementia. One explanation might be that the presence of cardiovascular risk factors, particularly present in patients with vascular dementia, may attenuate the positive effects of physical activity on cognition (Eggermont, Swaab, Luiten., & Scherder, 2006). The rationale is that during exercise, the blood supply to the muscles of patients with these risk factors occurs at the expense of the blood supply to e.g., the cerebrum. Consequently, the cognitive functioning of these patients might suffer rather than benefit from physical activity. For these patients, not the intensity of the physical activity but the variation in activities appears to be more important (Podewils et al., 2005).

Other studies confirm that, compared to older people without dementia, the level of aerobic physical activity and hence of physical energy expenditure is lower in Alzheimer patients (Pettersson, Engardt, & Wahlund, 2002; Poehlman et al., 1997), despite the fact that in one study 31.4% of the Alzheimer patients showed pacing behaviour (Wang et al., 2004).

Taken together, a decrease in the level of aerobic physical activity causes a decline in the level of physical activity energy expenditure, a relationship that with respect to dementia has so far only been examined in Alzheimer's disease and vascular dementia. In contrast to Alzheimer's disease, the risk for vascular dementia may not be reduced by physical activity, due to a prominent role of cardiovascular risk factors in its aetiology.

5.4 Conclusions

Studies that explore the relationship between ADL and hand motor activities, such as pouring a drink and handling coins, have so far been performed with cognitively intact older persons, but not with persons suffering from dementia. Most of the studies investigating the relationship between dementia and hand function are kinematic analyses that use digitizing tablets. It would be clinically relevant to examine the relationship between cognitive impairment and the performance of functional tasks in older persons with dementia, since these tasks represent ADL.

A decline in ADL due to an impaired hand motor function (Ranganathan et al., 2001a) might increase the risk of institutionalization (Ostwald et al., 1989).

Concerning gait I first conclude that gait disturbances are not preserved for the later stages of dementia but occur in the earliest stages and even in preclinical stages. In the second place, the nature of the disturbances in gait and gait-related motor disturbances appears to be closely related to the stage of the disease at which assessment takes place. Certain symptoms like impaired balance are most prominent in an early stage but disappear during the course of Alzheimer's disease (Dickin & Rose, 2004). In the third place, gait disturbances differ between the various stages and even in preclinical stages and may thus contribute to differential diagnosis. For example, apractic/ataxic gait has been observed in Alzheimer's disease but not in Mild Cognitive Impairment. In the fourth place, to draw the clinician's attention to gait disturbances as an important clinical feature of (preclinical) dementia, I propose a brief extension of the Mini-Mental State Examination (Folstein, Folstein, & Mchugh, 1975), by which gait can be rated from 0 (most disturbed) to 5 (normal) (see table 7). This rating is based on an existing rating scale developed to measure equilibrium and limb coordination (Franssen et al., 1999).

Test	Rating	Gait disturbance
6-m walk, turn,	5	Normal
6-m walk back,	4	Wide base, decreased velocity, decreased step length, static and
stand still,		dynamic instability, hesitation/freezing, reduced lower limb
lift up right foot (5 sec.),		strength (one bents a bit through the knees during walking)
lift up left foot (5 sec.)	3	4 + festination + head unsteadiness
	2	3 + rigidity, gait apraxia/ataxia, shuffling gait, bradykinesia
	1	2 + narrow base (instead of wide base)
	0	1 + stooped posture

Table 7. Assessment of gait and associated motor activity (rating based on the rating scale of Franssen et al., 1999). This item could be added to the Mini-Mental State Examination.

5.5 Questions

1. Which three types of hand motor function decline with aging?
2. Which finding supports the view that older persons are less able to coordinate the force of individual digits?
3. How do older persons compensate for a decline in precision-grip force?
4. Which hand motor function does not show a linear decline during aging?
5. Do older persons show compensatory activities in the brain during the performance of hand motor activity? Please elaborate.
6. Which hand motor activities show a difference between three groups, i.e., healthy controls, persons with Mild Cognitive Impairment, and patients with Alzheimer's disease (AD)?

7. Could you confirm the hypothesis that handwriting is associated with cognitive functioning? Please elaborate.

8. Which type of hand motor function has been examined in patients with vascular dementia? What was the effect of vascular dementia on this type of hand motor function?

9. Which neuronal network is associated with a precision-grip task and a sequence fist-edge-palm motor task?

10. Which network is associated with gross hand motor function such as motor speed?

11. What is meant by the 'last in – first out' phenomenon?

12. At which three levels can gait disorders be classified? Which part of the nervous system/brain areas/connections are associated with each separate level?

13. To which cognitive functions is higher level gait closely related?

14. Please explain the concept 'retrogenesis'. What is the clinical relevance of this concept?

15. For which subtypes of dementia, does the 'last in – first out' phenomenon hold for the SLF?

16. In what way does the SLF contribute to gait and gait-related motor activity?

17. Concerning the UF, does the 'last in – first out' phenomenon hold for one or more subtypes of dementia?

18. In what way does the UF contribute to gait and gait-related motor functions?

19. Does the 'last in – first out' phenomenon hold for the frontocerebellar connections? If so, for which subtype(s) of dementia?

20. Please address the contribution of the frontocerebellar connections to gait and gait-related motor functions.

21. For which subtype of dementia does the 'last in – first out' phenomenon concerning the frontostriatal network hold?

22. What are the consequences for gait in case of a dysfunction of frontostriatal connections?

23. With respect to the cingulum, the 'last in – first out' phenomenon applies to which two subtypes of dementia?

24. In which gait and gait-related motor functions is the cingulum involved?

25. Next to gait, also other factors may influence the level of physical activity. Which factors?

26. When in Alzheimer patients walking is combined with talking, which of these two functions will decline?

27. In what way do patients with vascular cognitive impairment no dementia have problems in motor activity and mood?

28. Does Subcortical ischaemic Vascular Dementia have an influence on IADL?

29. Please address the relationship between normal aging, aerobic physical activity, and energy expenditure?

30. What is the relationship between cardiovascular risk factors and energy expenditure?

31. Is there a relationship between leisure-time energy expenditure and risk of Alzheimer's disease?

32. Why might cardiovascular risk factors attenuate the positive effects of exercise on cognition in patients with dementia?

Chapter 6
Compensation and rehabilitation

6.1 Introduction

Aging of the brain is not a process that one undergoes passively and during which one can only wait for the cognitive deterioration to show up. There are both intrinsic and extrinsic strategies to limit the negative consequences of brain aging. From an intrinsic point of view, it is striking that the aging brain is able to activate compensatory strategies during the performance of cognitive tasks, maintaining its level as high as possible (Cabeza, Anderson, Locantore, & McIntosh, 2002). These compensatory strategies imply that brain areas that are activated during the performance of a certain task in elderly people are not 'switched-on' in young people performing the same task. In other words, specific neuronal functional circuits that are active in young people will not be the same active in elderly people performing the same task and vice versa. It is even more striking, that these intrinsic mechanisms have been observed in the brains of patients with dementia. Imagine, that despite the severe neuropathology affecting most cortical and subcortical areas, the brain is still capable of activating areas that are normally not involved in the execution of that specific function, as is the case in Alzheimer's disease (AD). These compensatory mechanisms will be presented first.

Although there is no cure for dementia, from an extrinsic point of view there are (non-)pharmacological interventions that may postpone the onset of dementia, reduce the risk for dementia, or attenuate its clinical consequences. For example, a non-pharmacological intervention such as an active lifestyle appears to have a beneficial influence on cognition in elderly people without dementia, by creating a 'cognitive reserve' that may protect against dementia. It is now known that dementia, irrespective of the subtype, coincides with motor disturbances such as disturbances in hand motor function and gait. Obtaining a lifestyle, as active as possible, requires optimal musculoskeletal functioning. Possibilities for rehabilitation of motor disturbances, including disturbances in hand motor function and gait disturbances, will be discussed in this chapter. The risk for dementia can also be reduced by an effective treatment of cardiovascular risk factors such as hypertension by non- pharmacological interventions such as exercise. Finally, studies examining effects of exercise on cognition of older persons with dementia and effects of cognitive training on the cognitive functions of older persons with dementia will be addressed in the final part of this chapter.

6.2 Compensatory strategies in aging and dementia

6.2.1 Elderly people without dementia: interhemispheric compensation

In a review, Cabeza (2002) indicates that elderly people show a bilateral rather than an unilateral activity in the prefrontal cortex (PFC) during the performance of a verbal memory task. The question arises whether bilateral activity reflects that the aging brain is still able to initiate compensatory strategies ('compensation hypothesis') or that it is a negative consequence of aging: the progressive disappearance of hemispheric asymmetry (difference between the left and right hemisphere) (Cabeza et al., 2002). To test both hypotheses, the activity of the PFC of three groups of elderly people was measured by means of PET, during the performance of a memory task. The three groups of elderly consisted of elderly persons who performed worse, elderly persons who performed well, and young adults (Cabeza et al., 2002). The results show that an increase in bilateral activity (or a decrease in hemispheric asymmetry) was observed in elderly with a high performance (see figure 1). Elderly persons with a low performance showed a hemispheric asymmetry that was similar to young people, albeit ineffective. It is suggested that elderly people with a low performance were not able to generate bilateral activity any more (Cabeza et al., 2002).

High-performing elderly people
without dementia

Low-performing elderly people
without dementia

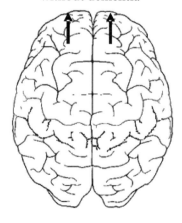 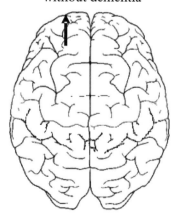

Figure 1. *Elderly people without dementia who show a high performance use bilateral PFC whereas low-performing elderly people without dementia are not able to initiate bilateral PFC activity. These results support the 'compensation hypothesis'. LH: left hemisphere; RH: right hemisphere.*

Referring to the former study, it has been claimed that PET is only able to assess an association between brain activity and test performance, and not a causal relationship (Rossi et al., 2004). An increase in activity in a specific area not necessarily indicates that that specific area is indeed involved in the execution of the task. A causal relationship can be demonstrated by means of repetitive Transcranial Magnetic Stimulation (rTMS). By means of rTMS it is possible to reduce the activity in one specific task-related area temporarily, causing a decline in test performance. In the rTMS study, a recognition memory task was administered to young people (age < 45 years) and elderly people (age > 50 years). It is argued that the left PFC plays a crucial role in encoding both verbal and nonverbal information and that the right PFC is important for the retrieval of information from memory. As mentioned before, lateralization as a compensatory mechanism reduces during aging. It has been observed that particularly the preference of the right PFC for the retrieval of information from memory reduces during aging and that the older person activates both hemispheres to compensate (Rossi et al., 2004). The preference of the left PFC for encoding showed no age effect.

In sum, the most important finding is that bilateral hemispheric activity represents a compensatory mechanism that is used by high-performing older people without dementia.

6.2.2 Elderly people without dementia: intrahemispheric compensation

A reduction in hemispheric asymmetry (or an increase in bilateral PFC activity) is not the only strategy elderly people use to perform cognitively as good as possible. During the performance of a task, brain areas of elderly people show an activity within a hemisphere (intrahemispheric) which they do not show in younger people. In a recent study, younger and older people had to remember photographs showing specific scenes such as a beach with palm trees (Gutchess et al., 2005). After a delay of 10 minutes, a recognition condition was administered. Functional MRI demonstrated that in elderly people the activity in the medial temporal lobe decreased, compensated by an increased activity in the PFC. The relationship between the activity in the medial temporal lobe and the PFC was even negative (see figure 2) (Gutchess et al., 2005).

The functional relationship between the hippocampus and the PFC, i.e., activity in the hippocampus coincides with activity in the PFC, is clearly demonstrated in a PET study (Grady, McIntosh, & Craik, 2003). During the scanning-procedure, young people and elderly persons had to remember objects and the names of these objects by means of a semantic strategy (choose between living or not living objects). In other words, the scans were made during the encoding of the information. During the performance of this task an increased activity was ob-

Right hemisphere
Elderly persons without dementia

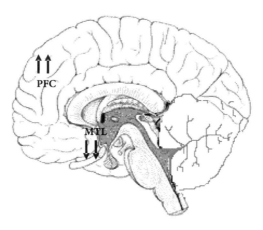

Figure 2. Intrahemispheric compensation in aging during the performance of a recognition memory task (Gutchess et al., 2005). During the performance of this task, activity in the medial temporal lobe (MTL) is decreasing (↓) in favour of an increased activity in the prefrontal cortex (PFC) (↑).

served in the anterior part of the hippocampus of all participants, irrespective of age. At the same time, however, activity was observed in the ventral frontal and occipitotemporal areas (perceptual processing of information) in the young participants whereas in the elderly people a combination with dorsal frontal and temporal areas (strategy selection) was found. The authors conclude that a well functioning recognition memory in elderly people depends on the combined activity of the dorsolateral PFC and the anterior part of the hippocampus.

Of note is that the nature of the stimulus determines which hemisphere (left or right) plays the major role: for recognition of objects the right hemisphere, for recognition of words the left hemisphere.

It is interesting that a transfer in activity of the amygdala-hippocampal system to the PFC has been observed in elderly persons during the performance of emotional memory tasks (Leigland, Schulz, & Janowsky, 2004). In that study, young and elderly people had to learn emotional (positive and negative) and neutral words and had to remember faces expressing all kinds of emotions. After a delay of 30 minutes, both groups remembered positive words better than neutral or negative words; similarly, both groups remembered positive and neutral faces better than faces with negative emotions. A subtle difference between both groups is that elderly people develop a better memory for positive emotions than for negative emotions which supports a transfer in the activity of the amygdala (negative emotions) to the activity of the PFC (positive emotions) (Leigland et al., 2004).

Yet, elderly do not always use the PFC for an optimal task performance; it depends on the nature of the task. Esposito and colleagues (1999) found age-related changes in the functional relationship between the PFC and the hippocampus during the performance of the Wisconsin Card Sorting Test (WCST) and the Raven Progressive Matrices (RPM). During the WCST, young people showed activity in the PFC combined with a decrease or even a lack of activity in the parahippocampal/hippocampal areas. However, in elderly people an increase in the (para) hippocampal activity together with a decrease in PFC activity was observed during the performance of the same task. During the performance of the RPM young people showed particularly activity in the parahippocampal/hippocampal areas and not in the PFC while elderly people showed a reversed pattern (Esposito, Kirkby, Van Horn, Ellmore, & Berman, 1999) (table 1).

	Young		Old	
	PFC	(Para)hippocampus	PFC	(Para)hippocampus
WCST	↑	↓	↓	↑
RPM	↑	↑	↑	–

Table 1. Intrahemispheric compensation in aging during the performance of the Wisconsin Card Sorting Test (WCST) and the Raven Progressive Matrices (RPM).

Taken together, the prefrontal cortex and the hippocampus are working closely together; in aging the PFC is able to increase its activity to compensate for an impaired activity in the medial temporal lobe. The PFC is particularly involved in positive emotions.

6.2.3 Compensation in elderly people with Mild Cognitive Impairment (MCI)

A 'plateau', i.e., a period of no change in cognitive impairment with a range of 3-6 years before the final diagnosis, has been observed in patients with Mild Cognitive Impairment (MCI) (Bäckman, Jones, Berker, Laukka, & Small, 2004). One of the explanations for this finding is that for a certain period of time, e.g., three years, the brain is able to compensate for the slowly progressing neuropathology. The neuropathology such as a loss of neurons will then reach a point at which compensatory mechanisms will fail and the cognitive impairment will become evident.

6.2.4 Alzheimer's disease: inter- en intrahemispheric compensation

Patients with Alzheimer's disease show bilateral activity in the PFC, similar to elderly with a normal mental status. However, in Alzheimer's disease the bilateral PFC activation coincides with a much larger activity in posterior brain regions.

This is in contrast to elderly people without dementia who showed a decrease in activity in posterior brain regions (e.g., the medial temporal lobe), in favour of the increased activity in the PFC (Gutchess et al., 2005).

Bilateral PFC activity in Alzheimer's disease should be considered as part of an extensive compensatory network (Grady et al., 2003). In one study, episodic and semantic memory tasks were administered to elderly people without dementia and patients with Alzheimer's disease (Grady et al., 2003). A remarkable finding was that in elderly without dementia the left ventrolateral PFC and temporal areas showed activity during the performance of the tasks whereas Alzheimer patients used bilateral PFC and bilateral temporoparietal activity for a correct performance of the task (see figure 3).

Elderly persons without dementia   Patients with Alzheimer's disease

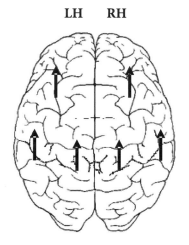

LH RH   LH RH

Figure 3. Intra- and interhemispheric compensation in patients with Alzheimer's disease during the performance of a task, compared to activity in brain areas of elderly persons without dementia. LH: left hemisphere; RH: right hemisphere.

It is emphasized that compensation in Alzheimer's disease concerns the whole network. Moreover, activity of this compensatory network appeared to be independent of the nature of the task: semantic or episodic; in other words, the compensatory network in Alzheimer's disease has a more global character.

The increased activity in posterior areas in Alzheimer patients during the performance of a task has also been found in other studies. In a PET study, the performance of elderly people without dementia on a verbal recognition task was compared with that of Alzheimer patients (Stern et al., 2000). The participants had to fulfil a simple task and a difficult task. Since the investigators succeeded in keeping the two levels of task load the same for both groups, it was possible to examine which functional neuronal circuits the two groups used to complete both the simple and difficult task. The PET data showed that during the execution of the difficult task with a high load on memory, elderly persons without dementia showed an increased activity in the left anterior cingulate cortex (attention during response-selection) and insula (top-down control of attention) (see figure 4).

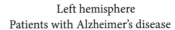

Left hemisphere
Elderly persons without dementia

Left hemisphere
Patients with Alzheimer's disease

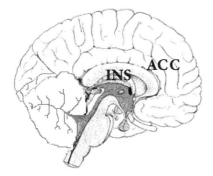
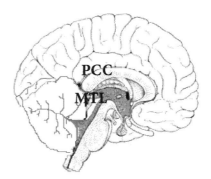

Figure 4. Performance of a difficult verbal recognition task by elderly people without dementia and patients with Alzheimer's disease. ACC: anterior cingulate cortex; PCC: posterior cingulate cortex; INS: insula; MTL: medial temporal lobe.

Patients with Alzheimer's disease activated more posterior brain areas such as the left posterior cingulate cortex and the left medial temporal cortex (see figure 4). These areas play an important role in the processing and encoding of words. Stern and colleagues (2000) suggest that this posterior perceptual network cooperates with memory-related circuits to improve the encoding and retrieval of information from memory. The PET-data further showed that the posterior network was also active in the elderly without dementia but this network did not show an increased activity during the difficult task.

In another study testing memory for faces for a somewhat longer time, patients with Alzheimer's disease showed a functional relationship between the left amygdala and the left PFC whereas controls showed a functional relationship between bilateral prefrontal cortices and the right hippocampus (Grady, Furey, Pietrini, Horwitz, & Rapoport,, 2001). The increased activity in the left amygdala in

Alzheimer patients, despite the known neuropathology in this area, supports compensatory mechanisms in Alzheimer's disease (see figure 5) (Grady et al., 2001).

In sum, independent on the nature of the task, patients with Alzheimer's disease initiate activity in the whole brain, both anterior and posterior, during the performance of a task. In other words, they use an extensive compensatory network.

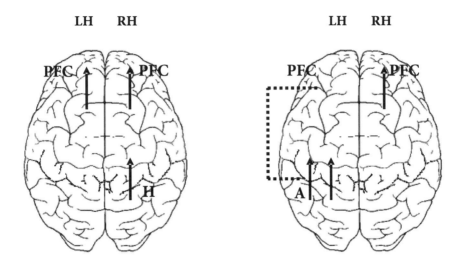

Figure 5. Functional relationship between bilateral prefrontal cortices (PFC) and the right hippocampus (H) in controls in remembering faces whereas patients with Alzheimer's disease showed a functional relationship between the left amygdala and the left PFC during the performance of the same task. LH: left hemisphere; RH: right hemisphere.

6.3 Rehabilitation of hand motor activity and gait in aging and dementia

6.3.1 Rehabilitation of hand motor dysfunction in aging and dementia

Hand motor dysfunction should be trained at a stage in which impairment and thus a decline in ADL might still be redressed. Indeed, training for pinch force, hand steadiness, and moving small objects has proven successful in healthy elderly people (Keogh, Morrison, & Barrett, 2006; Ranganathan, Siemionow, Sahgal, Liu, & Yue, 2001b). This is an important finding since many ADL tasks involve hand manipulation, and improvements in these areas could enhance quality of life (Ranganathan et al., 2001b). That said, not all aspects of the hand motor function are easy to train. For example, older people have more problems with releasing grip force, which is one aspect of the hand motor function that is not easy to train (Voelcker-Rehage & Alberts, 2005). This is unfortunate, since a decrease in releasing grip force plays a particularly important role in the impairment of hand function in older persons (Voelcker-Rehage & Alberts, 2005). Nevertheless, in older persons with a cognitive impairment, training of hand motor activity could still enhance the level of independence and perhaps postpone institutionalization. As far as I know, no clinical studies examining the effect of training on hand motor activity in dementia are available. Finally, future studies may show that each subtype of (preclinical) dementia has its own pattern of hand motor function impairment and therefore requires its own specific programme of rehabilitation.

6.3.2 Rehabilitation of gait disorders in dementia

Rehabilitation of gait disorders in dementia will be addressed as follows. The 'last in – first out' phenomenon (see Chapter 5) provides a theoretical basis for rehabilitation of gait and gait-related motor functions, functions that are vulnerable but still preserved or already affected in a mild stage of each subtype of dementia, i.e., Alzheimer's disease, frontotemporal dementia, and vascular dementia. These theoretical considerations will be discussed first. In addition, it is worthwhile to consider to what extent older persons with dementia are able to train gait-related motor functions, e.g., balance and muscle strength, in a non-pharmacological way. Finally, the relationship between pharmacotherapy and gait will be briefly highlighted.

'Last in – first out'; theoretical considerations for rehabilitation

Superior longitudinal fasciculus (SLF)
A disturbance in spatial awareness of limb and trunk might explain why patients in the early stages of Alzheimer's disease and vascular dementia display postural instability (table 2) (Scherder et al., 2007). Indeed, patients with Alzheimer's disease walk with a larger sway during the course of the disease (Nakamura et al., 1997). This strengthens the flow of sensory information and consequently contributes to postural control (Chen, Metcalfe, Chang, Jeka, & Clark, 2008). To prevent a further decline in or even to improve higher level gait, enhancement of body orientation and subsequently a decrease in sway might be achieved by, for example, touch and pressure (Jeka & Lackner, 1994). This technique might improve higher level gait and hence the level of physical activity in Alzheimer patients, as the primary somatosensory areas are relatively well-preserved (Kemppainen et al., 2006).

Five neuronal circuits	Contribution of five neuronal circuits to gait	Stage of structural maturation	Stage of structural degeneration and gait disturbances in dementia					
			AD		FTD		VaD	
			Stage of struct. degen.	Early gait disturbances	Stage of struct. degen.	Early gait disturbances	Stage of struct. degen.	Early gait disturbances
SLF	Awareness of limb and trunk location in body-centred space[1][†]	adulthood[2]	early[3]	Decrease in postural stability[4] Wide base[5]	early[6]	Involuntary trunk movements[7]	ns	Decrease in postural stability[8] Wide base[9]
UF	Imaging of sequences of foot movements[10]	adolescence[11]	early[12]	Decrease in steplength[13] and walking velocity[13]	early[6]		ns	Small step gait[14] Slow stepping[8] Apractic/ataxic gait[15]
Fronto-cerebellar connections	Coordination of limb movements[16]	childhood (Front/mot-med. crbl.)[17] adulthood (Inf front-lat. crbl.)[17]	ns		ns		ns	Unsteadiness[8]
	Upright posture[18][*]		ns	Dis-equilibrium[4]	ns		ns	
Frontostriatal connections	Spatial information necessary for gait[19] Movement initiation, planning[23]	adulthood[20]	late[21]		early[21]	Deficit in initiating motor activity[22]	ns	Start hesitation or freezing[9] Freezing upon turning[9]
Cingulum	Coordination, maintenance, and retrieval of complex foot movement sequences[24][25]	adulthood[26]	late[27]		early[28]		early[29]	Unsteadiness[8] Apractic[15]

Table 2 shows the role of five neuronal circuits in higher level gait and gait disturbances in early stage Alzheimer's disease (AD), vascular dementia (VaD), and frontotemporal dementia (FTD). The table also demonstrates in which subtype of dementia neuronal circuits mature late (adolescence/adulthood) and degenerate early (childhood) and vice versa ('last in – first out' phenomenon). The structural maturation stage and the stages of structural degeneration in the three subtypes of dementia that follow the 'last in – first out' phenomenon are highlighted yellow in the table. SLF: superior longitudinal fasciculus; UF: Uncinate fasciculus. Front/mot-med. crbl: primary, premotor, and supplementary cortices of the frontal lobe connected to the medial cerebellum; Inf front-lat. crbl.: inferior frontal gyrus and dorsolateral prefrontal cortex connected to the lateral cerebellum; ns=not studied; Stage of struct. degen.: stage of structural degeneration; *This function was not related to gait in the referred study; † study concerned monkeys.

[1]Schmahmann et al., 2007; [2]Giorgio et al., 2008; [3]Parente et al., 2008; [4]Nakamura et al., 1997; [5]O'Keeffe et al., 1996; [6]Borroni et al., 2007; [7]Mendez et al., 2005; [8]Pugh and Lipsitz, 2002; [9]Verghese et al., 2007a; [10]Jackson, Lafleur, Malouin, Richards, & Doyon, 2003; [11]Eluvathingal et al., 2007; [12]Taoka et al., 2006; [13]Goldman et al., 1999; [14]Tanaka et al., 1995; [15]Pohjasvaara et al., 2003; [16]Debaere et al., 2001; [17]Ridler et al., 2006; [18]Ouchi et al., 2004; [19]Bartels and Leenders, 2008; [20]Rubia et al., 2006; [21]Rabinovici et al., 2007; [22]de Mendonça et al., 2004; [23]Herrero et al., 2002; [24]Lafleur et al., 2002; [25]Heuninckx, Wenderoth, Debaere, Peeters, & Swinnen, 2005; [26]Dubois et al., 2006; [27]Naggara et al., 2006; [28]Barnes et al., 2007; [29]Stebbins et al., 2008.

The clinical consequence of the 'last in – first out' phenomenon for the gait-related motor functions of the separate brain regions belonging to the SLF is that the execution, initiation, planning, and selection of limb movements are vulnerable functions from the onset of frontotemporal dementia and vascular dementia in particular. These functions are less vulnerable in Alzheimer's disease due to, amongst others, the preservation of the premotor/supplementary motor cortex (Kemppainen et al., 2006). The loss of initiative in early stage frontotemporal dementia and vascular dementia implies that others should generate physical activity in the patients to prevent a further decline. The environment of, for example, a psychogeriatric ward, should stimulate the patients to move whenever they wish; in other words, it should be devoid of physical restraints (Cotter, 2005).

In addition, being related to the mirror-neuron system, the dorsolateral prefrontal cortex, the ventrolateral prefrontal cortex, and the inferior parietal lobe (table 3) show patterns of activation during the observation of gait and the imagination of initiating gait, walking, and walking with obstacles (Iseki, Hanakawa, Shinozaki, Nankaku, & Fukuyama, 2008; Malouin, Richards, Jackson, Dumas, & Doyon, 2003). The relatively well-preserved ventrolateral prefrontal cortex and mirror neurons specialized in foot movements (Binkofski & Buccino, 2006) in early stage Alzheimer's disease suggests that watching other people walk, for example, in a video, may enhance the patients' own ambulatory skills and prompt them to start walking again. This type of intervention is currently being studied in a group of patients with probable Alzheimer's disease. It should be noted that watching someone walk may not only activate the ventrolateral prefrontal cortex and premotor cortex but also the supplementary motor cortex (Wang, Wai, Kuo, Yeh, & Wang, 2008). The two latter areas are important for the preparation of gait, particularly when accompanied by a verbal cue such as 'ready' (Suzuki, Miyai, Ono, & Kubota, 2008). It is suggested that the motor system of Alzheimer patients may benefit from verbal commands during training sessions.

Uncinate fasciculus (UF)
The 'last in – first out' phenomenon holds for most of the UF-related areas (DLPFC, orbitofrontal cortex, (para) hippocampal region, ACC). One exception is the entorhinal cortex, which matures in childhood but is nevertheless affected in the early stages of all three subtypes of dementia ('last in – first out' phenomenon not applicable). Consequently, mental practising and imagination of foot movements should become a strategy for training the impaired motor representations related to higher level gait, from disease onset on, especially in a mild stage of vascular dementia; the orbitofrontal cortex, known for its motor imagery capacity (Jackson, Lafleur, Malouin, Richards, & Doyon, 2003) (table 3), is not as severely

Gait-related motor functions of brain regions belonging to the five neuronal circuits		Functional maturation-stage of gait-related motor functions			Stage of structural degeneration		
Frontal lobe	Gait-related motor functions*	Gait-related motor functions with maturation stage	Functional maturation stage	Structural maturation stage	AD	FTD	VaD
Primary motor cortex	Preparation and execution of movements[1]	Execution of walking[2]	childhood	childhood[3]	late[4]	late[5]	early[6]
Premotor/supplementary motor cortex	Execution, learning, initiation, planning, sequence, selection, and observation of movements[7,8,9]	Effect of observational modelling on movement[10]; Planning of movements[11,12]	childhood / childhood	childhood[3]	late[13]	early[14]	early[15]
Dorsolateral prefrontal cortex	Inhibitory motor control, motor imagery[16,17]	Action representation system/ motor imagery[18]; Motor inhibition[21]	adulthood / adolescence	adulthood[19]	early[20]	early[14]	early[15]
Ventrolateral prefrontal cortex	Imagery of foot movements[7]	Motor imagery[18]	adulthood	adulthood[22]	late[23]	early[24]	early[25]
Orbitofrontal cortex	Sequence of foot movements by motor imagery[26]	Motor imagery[18]	adulthood	adulthood[19]	early[27]	early[28]	early[6]
Parietal lobe							
Primary somatosensory areas	Sensori-motor integration[29]	Sensori-motor integration[30]	childhood	childhood[3]	late[4]	late[31]	early[15]
Superior parietal lobe	Imagination of standing and walking; imagination of precision gait; spatial navigation of leg movement[32,33]	Action representation system/ motor imagery[18]	adolescence	adolescence[3]	early[34]	early[34]	early[6]
Inferior parietal lobe	Executing sequential foot movements[35]; Observation and imagery of gait movement[41]	Decrease associated movements with age for alternating foot movements[36]; Observational modelling on movement dynamics[10]	adolescence / adulthood	adolescence/ adulthood[37]	early[38]	mid[39]	mid[40]
Superior temporal gyrus	Imagery and observation of standing, walking and running[42,43]	Action representation system/ motor imagery[18]	adolescence	adulthood[3]	early[44]	early[14]	early[45]
Entorhinal cortex; (para) hippocampal region	Spatial planning; navigation/ imagination of the environment[44,46,47]; Head direction and place cells/spatial navigation[51]	Spatial navigation[48]; Head- and trunk stabilization under normal vision[52]	adulthood / adulthood	childhood[3] / adulthood[53]	early[49] / early[54]	early[50] / early[14]	early[39] / early[45]
Occipital lobe							
Visual association areas	Visual input during bipedal locomotor activities[55]	Less dependent on visual information during maturation[56]	adulthood	ns	late[57]	early[58]	early[40]

	Motor function(s)	Gait-related function					
Striatum							
Caudate nucleus/putamen	Execution of well-learned sequence[47,59]; explicit and implicit learning of motor Sequences[60,59,62,63]; Balance[64]	Implicit visuomotor sequence learning[60]	adulthood	adolescence[61]	mid[66]	early[67]	early[15,68]
Thalamus	Motor and postural control[69]	Balance control[65]	adulthood	adolescence[61]	late[72]	early[5]	early[73]
Cingulum							
Anterior cingulate cortex	Gait[74]; Coordination complex foot movements[75]	Static standing balance[70]	childhood	childhood[71]	late[77]	early[78]	early[45]
Posterior cingulate cortex	Motor imagery of walking[17]	Stride-to-stride control of walking[76]; Action representation system/ motor imagery[30]	adolescence	adulthood[22]; adolescence[29]	early[80]	mid[78]	early[15]
Cerebellum	Timing and motor coordination lower extremities, including foot placement[81,82,83]	Lower limb coordination[84]	ns[a]	childhood[MCRB85] adulthood[LCRB85]	ns[a]	ns[a]	ns[a]

Table 3 Main gait-related motor functions of the *separate* brain areas belonging to the superior longitudinal fasciculus, uncinate fasciculus, frontocerebellar connections, frontostriatal connections, and cingulum, and stage of maturation. *Information extracted from animal experimental and human studies (healthy subjects and patients, irrespective of age). ns: not studied. ns[a]: concerning the functional maturation stage of gait-related motor functions and stage of structural degeneration, a distinction between medial and lateral cerebellum has not been made in literature. MCRB: medial cerebellum; LCRB: lateral cerebellum.

[1]Suzuki, Miyai, Ono, & Kubota; [2]Roncesvalles et al., 2000; [3]Cogtay et al., 2004; [4]Braak and Braak, 1991; [5]Diehl-Schmid et al., 2007; [6]Kerrouche et al., 2006; [7]Binkofski and Buccino, 2006; [8]Cunnington, Windischberger, & Moser, 2005; [9]Rushworth, Walton, Kennerley, & Bannerman, 2004; [10]Ashford, Davids, & Bennett, 2007; [11]Claxton, Keen, & McCarty, 2003; [12]von Hofsten, 2004; [13]Ouchi et al., 2004; [14]Berroni et al., 2007; [15]Grau-Olivares et al., 2007; [16]Kelly et al., 2004; [17]Malouin et al., 2003; [18]Choudbury, Charman, Bird, & Blakemore, 2007; [19]Segalowitz and Davies, 2004; [20]Kashani et al., 2008; [21]Rubia et al., 2000; [22]Eshe. et al., 2007; [23]Halliday, Double, Macdonald, & Kril, 2003; [24]Ibach et al., 2004; [25]Kuczynski, Jagust, Chui, & Reed, 2009; [26]Jackson et al., 2003; [27]Frisoni, Prestia, Rasser, Bonetti, & Thompson, 2009; [28]Nyatsanza et al., 2003; [29]Christensen et al., 2007; [30]Gasser, Rousson, Caflisch, & Largo, 2007; [31]Rosén, Gustafson, & Risberg, 1993; [32]Bakker et al., 2008; [33]Brown, Martinez, & Parsons, 2006; [34]Varrone et al., 2002; [35]Lafleur et al., 2002; [36]Gasser, Rousson, Caflisch, & Largo, 2007; [37]Olesen, Nagy, Westerberg, & Klingberg, 2003; [38]Kobayashi et al., 2008; [39]Du et al., 2007; [40]Stebbins et al., 2008; [41]Iseki, Hanakawa, Shinozaki, Nankaku, & Fukuyama, 2008; [42]Barraclough, 2008; [43]Jahn et al., 2004; [44]Lüth et al., 2005; [45]Shim, Yang, Kim, Shon, & Chung; [46]Sargolini et al., 2006; [47]Sheridan and Hausdorff, 2007; [48]Nardini, Jones, Bedford, & Braddick, 2008; [49]Hirao et al., 2006; [50]Richards et al., 2009; [51]Rolls, 1999; [52]Assaiante and Amblard, 1993; [53]Casey, Thomas, Davidson, Kunz, & Franzen, 2002; [54]Villain et al., 2008; [55]Fukuyama et al., 1997; [56]Vallis and McFadyen, 2005; [57]Meltzer et al., 1996; [58]Eslinger et al., 2007; [59]Jueptner et al., 1997; [60]Thomas et al., 2004; [61]Snook, Paulson, Roy, Phillips, & Beaulieu, 2005; [62]Floyer-Lea and Matthews, 2004; [63]Nakamura et al., 2001; [64]Rosano, Aizenstein, Studenski, & Newman, 2007; [65]Kirshenbaum, Riach, & Starkes, 2001; [66]Cousins et al., 2003; [67]Kim et al., 2007; [68]Yang et al., 2002; [69]Garcia-Cabezas, Rico, Sánchez-González, & Cavada, 2007; [70]Rival et al., 2005; [71]Zhang et al., 2005; [72]Luckhaus et al., 2008; [73]Kato et al., 2008; [74]Hanakawa et al., 1999; [75]Heuninckx et al., 2005; [76]Garcia-González, 2009; [77]Frisoni et al., 2007; [78]Barnes et al., 2007; [79]Marsh et al., 2006; [80]Parente et al., 2008; [81]D'Angelo and De Zeeuw, 2009; [82]Ivry, Keele, & Diener, 1988; [83]Stolze et al., 2002; [84]Cheron et al., 2001; [85]Ridler et al., 2006.

affected in vascular dementia as in Alzheimer's disease. Motor learning (grapho-motor task) by motor imagery appeared to be successful in patients with Huntington's Disease (HD) (Yágüez, Canavan, Lange, & Hömberg, 1999). The authors state that in a mild stage of Huntington's disease the cortical dopaminergic system, which is important for motor learning through motor imagery, is relatively intact. A deficit in the cortical dopaminergic system is not a neuropathological hallmark in a mild stage of vascular dementia, (Court & Perry, 2003) though the reverse applies in a mild stage of Alzheimer's disease and frontotemporal dementia (Kemppainen et al., 2006; Rinne et al., 2002).

Frontocerebellar connections
It should be borne in mind that the connections between inferior prefrontal cortex and (lateral) cerebellum mature late but are relatively well-preserved in a mild stage of Alzheimer's disease ('last in – first out' phenomenon not applicable) and thus provide opportunities for rehabilitation. In the first place, for those who are unable to take the initiative to start walking, moving the ankles in a passive way may coincide with activation of the primary, premotor and supplementary motor cortices, putamen, and cerebellum (Ciccarelli et al., 2005). These areas are important for preparing the sequence of foot movements and thus play a substantial role in higher level gait (Fukuyama et al., 1997; Sahyoun, Floyer-Lea, Johansen-Berg, & Matthews, 2004; Wang et al., 2008).

Next, the relatively well-preserved connection between the motor cortex and the cerebellum in mild Alzheimer's disease takes care of the timing of the separate components of complex motor activity (Diener & Dichgans, 1992). Such a programme would be particularly suitable for gait training as gait is a complex movement, which becomes even more complex when speed declines (Schablowski-Trautmann & Gerner, 2006). Training gait speed is clinically important as a decline in gait speed appears to be related to a decline in ADL (Potter, Evans, & Duncan, 1995); ADL, particularly executive functions, are dependent on cognitive functioning (Pereira, Yassuda, Oliveira, & Forlenza, 2008). Indeed, a linear relationship between a decline in gait speed and executive functions, such as working memory, has been observed in older persons over a period of five years (Inzitari et al., 2007). It is encouraging that older persons with mild to moderate dementia improved their scores for gait speed after six weeks of strength training of the lower limb muscles (Hageman & Thomas, 2002). Given the fore-mentioned results, it is not surprising that a slower walking speed is regarded as an early symptom of Alzheimer's disease (Pettersson, Olsson, & Wahlund, 2007).

Frontostriatal connections

The relative intactness of the striatum as part of the dorsolateralprefrontal cortex-striatum connection in Alzheimer's disease (contesting the 'last in – first out' phenomenon) explains why implicit, automatic motor learning is the most appropriate type of motor learning in Alzheimer's disease (van Halteren-van Tilborg, Scherder, & Hulstijn, 2007). It is less known that the same system may contribute to explicit motor learning in Alzheimer's disease, for example, by explicit training of stride length which is reduced in Alzheimer's disease (Scherder et al., 2007). Constant training is, however, essential in order to automate the task (Dick, Hsieh, Dick-Muehlke, Davis, & Cotman, 2000). This implies a novel approach in rehabilitation as most intervention studies aimed at improving higher level gait use interventions that take place, for example, three times a week for a limited period (Lazowski et al., 1999).

Cingulum

In a mild stage of Alzheimer's disease neuropathology is particularly present in the PCC and not in the ACC and vice versa in frontotemporal dementia; this might explain why topographic orientation is relatively spared in mild frontotemporal dementia and not in mild Alzheimer's disease (Grossi et al., 2002). However, frontotemporal dementia patients who are carriers of apolipoprotein ε4 show hypoperfusion in the parahippocampal region (Borroni et al., 2006). As the parahippocampal region is connected to the PCC and thus plays a role in mental navigation (Mellet et al., 2000), hypoperfusion makes topographic orientation vulnerable. Therefore, it might be beneficial to assign route-learning tasks to frontotemporal dementia patients from the onset of the disease.

The relatively well-preserved visuospatial capacity in frontotemporal dementia might offer another strategy for training higher level gait (Barnes et al., 2007; Kertesz, Blair, McMonagle, & Munoz, 2007), which might enable patients to imagine standing and walking upright (PCC). For example, a programme could start with videos of walking persons (third-person perspective), followed by videos shot from a first-person perspective. Persons with and without higher level gait disturbances could be presented in both videos and the patients could be trained in observing the differences. Such a programme might help patients to maintain or correct their own gait.

Furthermore, the relative intactness of areas such as the ACC, together with the striatum in mild to moderate Alzheimer's disease (Halliday, Double, Macdonald, & Kril, 2003; Herholz, 2003), implies that these patients should be afforded the opportunity to explicitly practise over-learned motor activity such as walking and other (instrumental) ADL ((I)ADL). Such an approach requires a revolutionary change in nursing home care as the current lifestyle of many nursing home residents is characterized by inactivity and long periods spent in bed (Alessi & Schnelle, 2000; Kolanowski, Buettner, Litaker, & Yu, 2006). A small homelike care unit might constitute the type of environment that invites patients with dementia to participate in (I)ADL (Verbeek, van Rossum, Zwakhalen, Kempen, & Hamers, 2009).

Conclusions

The present findings suggest that the 'last in – first out' phenomenon, also implying that neuronal circuits or brain regions that mature early are less vulnerable for neurodegenerative disease, may provide new strategies for the prevention of upcoming higher-level gait disturbances and for the rehabilitation of already present higher level gait disturbances; albeit for Alzheimer's disease, frontotemporal dementia and vascular dementia in a different way. Even if the 'last in – first out' phenomenon is not applicable, strategies for the rehabilitation of higher level gait can be developed.

Alzheimer's disease. The majority of the new therapeutic strategies are applicable for patients in a mild stage of Alzheimer's disease in particular. For example, for those Alzheimer patients who are ambulatory but do not take the initiative to walk anymore, passive ankle movements (frontocerebellar connections) and watching videos of walking people (SLF; cingulum) may be of value. In mild Alzheimer patients implicit and explicit training of complex over-learned motor activity such as gait (speed) (frontocerebellar and frontostriatal connections, cingulum) is possible as long as the training is applied regularly over a longer period, and the environment, for example, a small home-like care unit, permits this type of activation. If there are higher level gait disturbances, increased sway for example, light touch on e.g., a bar by the patient (SLF) might improve this disorder.

Frontotemporal dementia. Similar to mild Alzheimer's disease, in mild frontotemporal dementia patients' ambulatory skills may react positively to watching walking from both third- and first-person perspectives on videos (SLF). Furthermore, to prevent topographic disorientation in frontotemporal dementia patients (cingulum), route learning could be a valuable intervention.

Vascular dementia. For mild vascular dementia patients, dancing is one strategy to prevent or improve higher level gait disturbances. After dancing, these patients might be able to imagine the steps just learned, and hence improve locomotion (UF).

Taken together, there are several strategies for rehabilitation of higher level gait and gait-related motor activity in dementia; with for each subtype of dementia a different approach. Nevertheless, the majority of rehabilitation strategies to improve higher level gait and gait-related motor activity in patients with dementia have failed. In these studies, patients with mild to severe dementia are included, without further specification of the subtype of dementia (Hageman & Thomas, 2002; Littbrand, Lundin-Olsson, Gustafson, & Rosendahl, 2009; Netz, Axelrad, & Argov, 2007; Pomeroy et al., 1999; Thomas & Hageman, 2003). The negative findings reported by these studies are observed irrespective of the nature of the training programme (mobility, strength, balance or a combination of these aspects), the duration per treatment session (30-45 minutes), the number of treatment sessions (10-30) and duration of the treatment period (6-12 weeks). The negative findings have been explained by a too short intervention period (e.g., 6 weeks; Littbrand et al., 2009) and a too low intensity of the programme, e.g., exercise while sitting (Netz et al., 2007; Hageman & Thomas, 2002).

I argue that in addition to these above-mentioned explanations, also the subtype of the dementia plays a role in the outcome of the rehabilitation programme. The rationale underlying this suggestion is that most therapeutic strategies are applicable for patients in a mild stage of Alzheimer's disease in particular. Indeed, in a recent randomized block design study, mild to moderate Alzheimer patients showed an improvement in lower limb strength, flexibility, dynamic balance, endurance fitness, and gait after a 12-week training programme, performed 3 times a week, for approximately 75 minutes per session (Santana-Sosa, Barriopedro, López-Mojares, Pérez, & Lucia, 2008). These results should be considered with caution, given the small number of participants in each group (8); the effect sizes, however, were large. Similarly, in mild to moderate Alzheimer patients, an improvement in lower limb strength by a training programme consisting of aerobic fitness, strength training, and training of balance/flexibility showed a trend (Steinberg, Leoutsakos, Podewils, & Lyketsos, 2009). Unfortunately, effect sizes were not calculated. The question whether the effectiveness of a rehabilitation programme depends on its content in relation to the specific subtype of dementia cannot be answered yet and requires extensive further research.

The present results further show that rehabilitation strategies based on functions that are relatively preserved in the three subtypes of dementia are not unlimited. Consequently, at a very mild stage of dementia, one should focus on training higher level gait and gait-related motor functions which are bound to be disturbed in the near future. For each subtype of dementia, this approach provides clear indications about which functions are most vulnerable. On the other hand, the motor functions described above emerge mainly from the cooperation between several brain regions within a specific network. However, the different brain regions belonging to one or more of the five neuronal networks may have their own roles in higher level gait and gait-related motor functions. These higher level gait and gait-related motor functions are presented in table 3 and create further opportunities for rehabilitation for each subtype of dementia, taken the neuropathology as shown in figures 2-4 (chapter 5) into consideration.

Training gait-related motor disturbances in dementia

Next to a differential diagnostic value, the specific nature of the gait disturbances should be treated by an exercise programme that is focused on that specific disturbance. This line of research has received little attention so far. In some studies a more 'general' exercise programme was applied. For example, an exercise programme accompanied by music was presented to late stage Alzheimer patients who showed an improved balance after the treatment period (Francese, Sorrell, & Butler, 1997). In another study, a programme consisting of walking and riding an exercise bicycle improved dynamic and static balance in Alzheimer patients (Rolland et al., 2000). Only a few studies examined the possibility to train specific gait-related elements, such as (dynamic) balance, in dementia. In one study with elderly people with dementia and a history of falling, walking, flexibility and static balance reacted positively to a physical activity programme which included exercises that were specifically focused on these dependent variables (Toulotte, Fabre, Dangremont, Lensel, & Thevenon, 2003). Specific balance training appeared to be possible in one study (Dickin & Rose, 2004), but could not be replicated in another study (Chong, Horak, Frank, & Kaye, 1999). However, in the latter study, the level of cognitive function of the Alzheimer patients showed a large variation, i.e., MMSE scores ranged from 8-27. As far as I know, effects of training specific aspects of gait and/or gait-related motor activity in other subtypes of (preclinical) dementia has not been studied.

In sum, the few studies so far suggest that balance is a gait-related motor disturbance that can be trained. In a recent systematic review, Blankevoort and co-workers (2010) add that next to balance, also gait speed, functional mobility, and lower-extremity strength can be trained in patients with dementia, irrespective of the stage of dementia. Moreover, the authors found that in particular multicomponent interventions were the most effective, i.e., interventions combining strength, endurance, and flexibility.

Pharmacotherapy for parkinsonian and higher-level gait symptoms

Differentiating between parkinsonian (basal ganglia) and higher-level (subcortical and cortical) symptoms may yield interesting suggestions for treatment (Kurlan, Richard, Papka, & Marshall, 2000). For example, Alzheimer's disease is characterized by both parkinsonian and higher-level gait symptoms such as slowness in walking and impaired balance (O'Keeffe et al., 1996; Goldman, Baty, Buckles, Sahrmann, & Morris, 1999; Alexander et al., 1995; Pettersson et al., 2002; Sheridan et al., 2003). As far as I know, studying the effects of L-Dopa on the parkinsonian signs in Alzheimer's disease has not taken place so far, but might be a challenging future goal. Furthermore, it has been suggested that cholinesterase inhibitors may improve higher-level gait disturbances by enhancing cortical cholinergic degeneration instead of basal ganglia degeneration (Hutchinson & Fazzini, 1996). Support for this latter suggestion emerges from studies in which the hand movements of Alzheimer patients were examined. In mild to moderate Alzheimer patients, simple hand motor activity was performed much slower than in controls (Babiloni et al., 2000). EEG recordings showed hyperactivity in areas adjacent to the primary motor cortex i.e., the frontomedial and ipsilateral Rolandic cortical areas. These areas might become hyperactive by a decrease in inhibition which is caused by a decline in the functional connectivity between the temporal, parietal, occipital, and frontal areas. It has been suggested that this functional disconnection is due to a dysfunction of the cholinergic pathways that connect these areas (Babiloni et al., 2004). The effect of a cholinergic deficit on the frontomedial cortex is particularly interesting since a strong association between a dysfunction of the frontomedial cortex, in particular the supplementary motor area, and gait apraxia has been described (Della Sala, Francescani, & Spinnler, 2002).

Since cholinesterase inhibitors appeared to provoke parkinsonian symptoms in Alzheimer's disease (Trabace et al., 2000), it was interesting to review recent studies examining the effects of cholinesterase inhibitors on motor activity in Parkinsons's disease. In two studies, Physostigmine and Rivastigmine aggravated parkinsonian signs in Parkinson's disease (Werber & Rabey, 2001; Richard, Justus, Greig, Marshall, & Kurlan, 2002). In another study, Galanthamine reduced Parkinsonism in 6 out of 13 patients but aggravated Parkinsonism in 3 patients (Aarsland, Mosimann, & McKeith, 2003). Moreover, from the original group of 16 patients, 1 patient dropped out due to an increase in tremor. An explanation for these equivocal results might be that, similar to Alzheimer's disease, in Parkinson patients motor disturbances are of both parkinsonian and higher-level nature (Rossini, Filippi, & Vernieri, 1998). By improving the latter, cholinesterase inhibitors may contribute to an 'overall clinical improvement' in Parkinsonism.

In sum, the effects of cholinesterase inhibitors should be examined on higher-level gait and gait-related motor activity in Alzheimer's disease and not only with respect to cognition, as has been done so far. To evaluate the effects of cholinesterase inhibitors on motor activity in Parkinson's disease, a distinction should be made between parkinsonian and higher-level symptoms.

6.3.3 Cardiovascular risk factors, dementia, and treatment

White matter lesions play an important role in the development of dementia, both Alzheimer's disease and vascular dementia (Schmidt, Schmidt, & Fazekas, 2000). White matter lesions, a reflection of cerebral microangiopathy, damage fronto-subcortical connections resulting in cognitive disturbances such as a decline in executive functions, mobility, balance, and mood (Pugh & Lipsitz, 2002). White matter lesions, particularly periventricular white matter lesions, and grey matter lesions are strongly related to cardiovascular risk factors (Pugh & Lipsitz, 2002; Schmidt et al., 2000). Cardiovascular risk factors for both Alzheimer's disease and vascular dementia include obesity, arterial hypertension, diabetes mellitus, atrial fibrillation, atherosclerosis, and smoking (Schmidt et al., 2000). Particularly cardiovascular risk factors initiate a cascade of events in which degenerative processes cause a decrease in metabolism, with a subsequent decline in cerebral perfusion. A decline in cerebral perfusion coincides with white and grey matter lesions, and brain atrophy (Meyer, Rauch, Rauch, Haque, & Crawford, 2000). In this way, cardiovascular risk factors may eventually lead to dementia (figure 6) (Luchsinger & Mayeux, 2004).

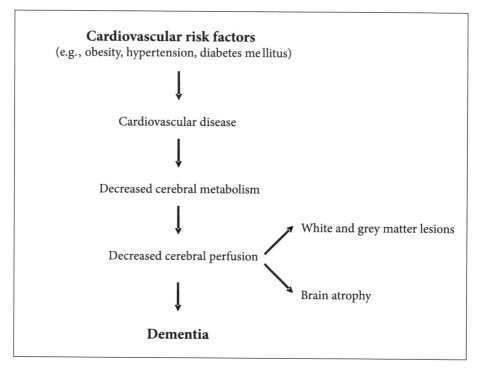

Figure 6. Cascade of events, initiated by cardiovascular risk factors, finally resulting in dementia.

It has been observed that the risk for white matter lesions increased 20-fold in case of hypertension that existed 20 years or longer, particularly in elderly persons aged between 60-70 years (de Leeuw et al., 2002). Hypertension but also diabetes mellitus are strongly related to overweight (obesity). More specifically, obesity is the basis for a metabolic disorder that is responsible for hypertension, congestive heart failure, and insulin resistance leading eventually to cardiovascular disease (Sharma & Chetty, 2005). Insulin resistance not only contributes to cardiovascular disease, it also brings about a decrease in glucose tolerance, hyperglycaemia, and finally type 2 diabetes ('insulin resistance syndrome') (Rao, 2001; Sharma & Chetty, 2005). Consequently, diabetes and cardiovascular disease are closely related. Dagres and colleagues (2004) examined the relationship between insulin resistance and the reactivity of coronary arteries in adults with chest pain. They observed that insulin sensitivity is related to vasoreactivity in the coronary arteries, i.e., the higher the insulin sensitivity, the larger the coronary vasoreactivity (Dagres et al., 2004). The rationale is that insulin contributes to vasodilatation by means of nitric oxide which is released from the endothelium in the wall of blood vessels (Verma et al., 2001). Patients who are insulin resistant show an impairment in nitric oxide mediated vasodilatation (Reusch, 2002), causing vasoconstriction and hypertension. Hypertension also coincides with an increase in neurofibrillary tangles and amyloid plaques in Alzheimer's disease (Schmidt et al., 2000) (figure 7). Control of these risk factors is essential for maintaining optimal cognitive functioning.

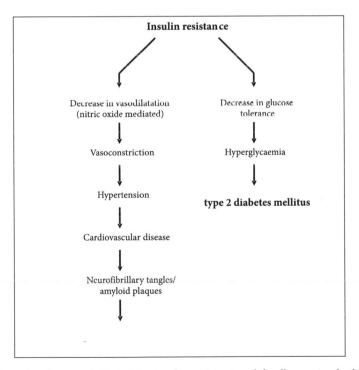

Figure 7. Cascade of events, initiated by insulin resistant and finally causing both Alzheimer's disease and type 2 diabetes mellitus.

It will take some time however before cardiovascular risk factors cause ischemic cerebral microangiopathy (e.g., white matter lesions). Therefore, it is important to treat cardiovascular risk factors like hypertension as soon as possible, a treatment that should include medications, changes in dietary and lifestyle among which physical activity (Reuter-Lorentz, & Lustig, 2005). Within the scope of this book, the influence of lifestyle on cardiovascular risk factors will be discussed in more detail.

Medication

It is not illogical that the influence of hypertension on white matter depends on the success of its treatment. In one study it has been observed that those who were treated for hypertension but did not show the expected effect, i.e., despite the medication they still had a systolic blood pressure > 140 mmHG and a diastolic blood pressure > 90 mmHG, showed more white matter lesions than untreated hypertensives (Liao et al., 1996). Although this may seem odd at first sight, an explanation for this latter finding is that the increased blood pressure was probably not high enough to require medication and therefore had a lesser impact on white matter (Liao et al., 1996).

Dietary

A direct relationship between obesity and hypertension has been described above (Sharma & Chetty, 2005). In a recent study, the effects of a diet that included fruit, vegetables, and low-fat dairy products (called DASH: Dietary Approaches to Stop Hypertension) on hypertension was examined (Nowson et al., 2005). The effects of the DASH diet were compared to the effects of another low-fat diet. The difference between both diets was that the DASH-diet included advices about quantity and frequency of the intake of e.g., fruit and vegetables whereas the low-fat diet only emphasized that one should take more fruit and vegetables (for more details, see Nowson et al., 2005). It should be noted however that the diet was combined with a physical activity program and that in both groups also people using antihypertensive medication were included. The results show that the participants of both groups showed a comparable weight loss. Those who took the DASH diet showed larger decreases in both systolic and diastolic blood pressure, but the mechanism underlying this finding remains unclear (Nowson et al., 2005).

Considering the fact that obesity, and hence high hypertension, are closely related to a decrease in insulin sensitivity (Sharma & Chetty, 2005), it was examined in a recent study whether a program of among others the DASH-diet plus physical activity would exert a beneficial influence on insulin sensitivity (Ard et al., 2004). The results show that insulin sensitivity increased, together with weight loss. In other words, this program improved insulin action and, consequently, reduced cardiovascular disease risks.

Lifestyle

In a review, it was demonstrated that in elderly people an active lifestyle is strongly associated with a higher level of cognitive functioning (Fratiglioni, Paillard-Borg, & Winblad, 2004). Considering the fact that most studies are cross-sectional, the direction of this relationship is not clear (Newson & Kemps, 2005). They pose the question whether people who are cognitively better, are also more interested in physical activity or whether an engagement in 'activity' improves cognitive functioning. Newson and Kemps (2005) examined the relationship between an active lifestyle that is so general that it approaches the daily activities as close as possible, in a combined cross-sectional and a 6-year longitudinal study. Data from the cross-sectional analyses revealed a clear association between this general lifestyle activities and cognitive functions such as speed of information processing, picture naming, implicit memory, and verbal fluency. Longitudinal data-analyses showed that general lifestyle activities positively influenced changes in the performance on the same neuropsychological tests, except for verbal fluency. Changes in verbal fluency during this period were completely related to sensory function, i.e., hearing and vision (Newson & Kemps, 2005).

An active lifestyle can also be subdivided into social, mental, and physical activity (Fratiglioni et al., 2004). The finding that a rich social environment decreases the risk of death (Fratiglioni et al., 2004) could be explained as follows. A decline in the social environment may provoke cardiovascular disease and stroke (Fratiglioni et al., 2004), damaging the physical condition, and increasing the risk of death. In line with these findings is that social support may be one of the mechanisms that plays an essential role in the recovery after stroke (Fratiglioni et al., 2004). With respect to mental activity, irrespective of whether the activity takes place in a group or alone, people live longer when they are engaged in all kinds of leisure activities such as singing in a choir or reading books (Fratiglioni et al., 2004). These latter activities stimulate cognitive processes, resulting in a 'cognitive reserve' (Fratiglioni et al., 2004) that may delay the onset of e.g., Alzheimer's disease. This 'cognitive reserve' hypothesis or 'brain reserve' hypothesis has also been brought forward with respect to the effects of education on cognitive aging (Kramer, Bherer, Colcombe, Dong, & Greenough, 2004). A high level of education could prevent cognitive decline during aging because education has a beneficial influence on the development of neuronal networks. Compared to networks that are not stimulated by education, the enhanced neuronal networks are better able to face the neuropathological and functional consequences of aging. Indeed, studies have shown that low levels of education increase the risk for Alzheimer's disease.

Also in non-demented elderly persons, low education was related to white matter lesions and cerebral atrophy (Kramer et al., 2004). They further emphasize that there is no consensus about the direction of this relationship: do people with an initial large brain capacity automatically go for the highest level of education or is a large brain capacity really the result of a high level of education. Support for the latter assumption arises from studies that show that elderly persons are still able to learn specific cognitive skills, although the complexity of the information to be processed may limit the training effects (Kramer et al., 2004). Moreover, the improvement in cognitive skills was not reflected in an improvement in activities of daily life. The fact that learned skills cannot be generalized to activities of daily life, may weaken the 'cognitive reserve' hypothesis and rather point to a benefit of the training in that specific field (Kramer et al., 2004). The third ingredient of an active lifestyle is physical activity that will be discussed in more detail in the next section.

6.3.4 Physical activity, cardiorespiratory fitness, and cognition

The risk for cardiovascular disease and mortality in sedentary men with diabetes mellitus is increased by low cardiovascular fitness (Reusch, 2002). Sedentary lifestyle in patients with diabetes might be due to insulin resistance (see above). In addition, reduced maximal oxygen consumption (VO2max) is characteristic for patients with type 2 diabetes (Reusch, 2002). However, compared to women with overweight and leanness, women with type 2 diabetes showed the largest increase in exercise capacity.

A number of studies indicate the beneficial influence of exercise on the cardiovascular condition, diabetes, hypertension, obesity, and insulin resistance (Mazzeo & Tanaka, 2001). Irrespective of type, intensity, and duration of the intervention, and irrespective of pre-treatment blood pressure and the use of antihypertensive drugs, aerobic exercise reduces the blood pressure in hypertensive patients (Stewart, 2002). More specifically, walking as an intervention during 25 weeks lowered systolic and diastolic blood pressure by 3 and 2 mmHG, respectively (Stewart, 2002). Regular aerobic exercise reduces the storage of adipose tissue, specifically in the upper body (Mazzeo & Tanaka, 2001). As mentioned before, insulin resistance in diabetes mellitus is strongly associated with an impairment in nitric oxide mediated vasodilatation, also in the coronary arteries, resulting in cardiovascular disease (Stewart, 2002). Stress on the endothelium of the vessel wall, caused by exercise, stimulates the release of nitric oxide, and thus vasodilatation (Stewart, 2002). This mechanism underlies the increase in vasoreactivity in the forearm of type 2 diabetes patients (Stewart, 2002). In hypertensive patients, brisk walking enhanced the release of nitric oxide and decreased the systolic and diastolic blood pressure by 8 and 4 mmHG (Stewart, 2002). Nitric oxide itself regulates the release of tissue-type plasminogen activator (t-PA) (Schini-Kerth, 1999), an enzyme that plays a crucial role in preventing thrombosis and in degrading fibrin clots in the circulation (Muldowney & Vaughan, 2002; Lijnen & Collen, 1997).

Cardiorespiratory fitness is particularly enhanced by aerobic exercises (Colcombe et al., 2004). It has been observed that aerobic and not anaerobic activity is a necessary condition for improving cognition. Kramer and colleagues (1999) examined the effect of walking (aerobic) and stretching/toning (anaerobic) on executive functions of healthy sedentary elderly. Improvement in executive functions was only observed after walking which coincided with a significant increase in the maximum rate of oxygen consumption. They conclude that specifically those executive functions improved that were mediated by the PFC. It has been suggested that an increase in cardiovascular fitness by e.g., walking for 6 months, enhances brain plasticity in elderly persons (Colcombe et al., 2004). The results are of great clinical importance since they show that moderate physical activity improves prefrontal cortex functioning and, consequently, independent functioning (Colcombe et al., 2004). The question whether the improvement in cognitive functioning by exercise is indeed mediated by an improvement in cardiorespiratory function, cannot be answered yet (Angevaren, Aufdemkampe, Verhaar, Aleman, & Vanhees, 2008).

6.3.5 Physical activity and cognition in (preclinical) dementia; intervention studies

The number of studies examining the effects of exclusively exercise, i.e., not combined with for example music, on cognition in older persons with dementia is increasing. In only one very early study, 'geriatric mental patients' participated in an exercise programme; these patients showed improved logical reasoning and memory performance compared to a control group (Powell, 1974). In a more recent study, an exercise programme consisting of walking with a rollator resulted in improved executive functioning in older people with Mild Cognitive Impairment compared with a control group that received social visits (Scherder et al., 2005). However, the number of patients in each group was relatively small (n = 15). A much larger number of patients at risk for Alzheimer's disease (n = 138) participated in a randomized controlled trial in which the persons in the experimental group participated in a home-based physical activity programme (Lautenschlager et al., 2008). Cognitive functioning, among which word list recall, improved after the treatment period of 18 months.

The question arises whether physical activity (exercise) is also beneficial for cognitive functioning in patients diagnosed with dementia. Findings appear to be inconsistent. For example, Alzheimer patients who participated in a walking programme showed improved communication compared with patients that followed a conversation programme (Friedman & Tappen, 1991). A programme of somatic and isotonic-relaxation exercises in which Alzheimer patients participated led to improved cognitive abilities compared with a control group (Lindenmuth & Moose, 1990). Unfortunately, the participants were not randomly assigned to the experimental or control group and they did not participate in the exercises regularly. In one study Alzheimer patients exercised on a cyclo-ergometer. After the treatment period, short-term memory and global mental functioning were found to be improved (Palleschi et al., 1996). Global mental functioning of another group of Alzheimer patients was also found to be improved after an exercise programme that consisted of walking and cycling on an ergometer (Rolland et al. 2000). Unfortunately, a control group was lacking in both studies. Results of recent randomized controlled trials including patients in a more advanced stage of dementia, a 6-week walking programme did not have a beneficial effect on cognitive functioning (Eggermont, Swaab, Hol, & Scherder, 2009). One of the explanations might be the high prevalence of cardiovascular diseases (Eggermont et al., 2009). Cardiovascular risk factors, cerebral perfusion and hence cognition could rather decrease instead of increase during aerobic physical activity. In other words, exercise programmes should be applied with caution.

In sum, effects of exercise on cognition in people with (preclinical) dementia are inconsistent. In addition, as a reaction to exercise training, older participants may lower down their spontaneous activity in the non-training period (Westerterp, 2000). In such cases, there will be hardly any profit from exercise-training. Furthermore, a physical activity program should take into consideration the specific gait and gait-related motor deficits that accompany (preclinical stages) of dementia. Only then, a physical activity program can reach its highest level of effectiveness on physical functioning and consequently on cognition. Finally, physical activity as an intervention to stabilize or even improve cognitive functioning in older people with (preclinical) dementia should be applied as early as possible. The assumption that even small changes in gait or in gait-related motor activity may initiate the onset of a decrease in the level of physical activity and hence in cognition, warrants further research.

6.3.6 Biological mechanisms underlying social, mental, and physical activity

The social, mental, and physical activity could be considered as a type of 'enriched environment' of which common underlying mechanisms include synaptogenesis, vascular plasticity, i.e. angiogenesis, and neurogenesis (Churchill et al., 2002).

Synaptogenesis implies that the level of neuropil shows a positive correlation with the level of complexity of the environment (Churchill et al., 2002). The brain of an animal that together with other animals lives in a cage filled with toys ('enriched environment') responds more positively, i.e., heavier and thicker cortex, than the brain of an animal that lives solitary ('impoverished'). Synaptogenesis not only takes place in the cerebral cortex but also in the cerebellum, and is therefore not dependent on a specific brain region (Churchill et al., 2002). A prerequisite for synaptogenesis is that one has to learn a specific task, otherwise synaptogenesis will not occur. A second mechanism underlying the effects of enriched environment is angiogenesis (Churchill et al., 2002). As a response to exercise and enriched environment, already existing blood vessels produce new capillaries. Similar to synaptogenesis, angiogenesis can take place all over the brain (e.g., cerebellum, primary motor cortex) and during the whole life span. Angiogenesis is not a static process but a phenomenon that is able to adjust to more demanding situations like exercise (Churchill et al., 2002).

In addition to synaptogenesis and angiogenesis, the brain is also able to add new neurons. This process is called neurogenesis and takes place in, for example, the hippocampus (Churchill et al., 2002; Fossati, Radtchenko, & Boyer, 2004). Neurotransmitters like serotonin and neurotrophins like brain-derived neurotrophic factor (BDNF) respond to exercise and may contribute to cell proliferation (neurogenesis). The finding that an enriched environment improves learning and locomotor activity reflects that brain plasticity, induced by enriched environment, can be maintained over a longer period (Fossati et al., 2004). In contrast, cell proliferation decreases in the presence of stress which itself enhances the release of corticosteroids.

Taken together, cardiovascular risk factors, particularly hypertension, are strongly related to white and grey matter lesions. Obesity is one of the causes of hypertension but also of type 2 diabetes mellitus, another cardiovascular risk factor. Type 2 diabetes mellitus itself might contribute to hypertension. Hypertension might be responsible for the neuropathology in Alzheimer's disease such as plaques and tangles. Therefore, hypertension must be treated as early as possible by medications, and changes in dietary and lifestyle in which physical activity plays a major role. Several mechanisms underlie the positive effects of walking on hypertension and type 2 diabetes mellitus, among which nitric oxide. The beneficial effects of physical activity on cognition may be explained by synaptogenesis, angiogenesis, and neurogenesis.

6.3.7 Cognitive training in aging and dementia

The results of a recent Cochrane review clearly show that there is no scientific evidence for an effect of training on cognitive functions of healthy older persons and persons with Mild Cognitive Impairment (Martin, Clare, Altgassen, Cameron, & Zehnder, 2011). A few years earlier, Clare and Woods (2003) reviewed studies concerning the effects of cognitive training in early stage Alzheimer's disease and vascular dementia. No firm conclusions about the effectiveness of cognitive training in these two populations can be drawn, as randomized controlled trials are missing. In a more recent review, various types of cognitive training were described as effective in improving cognitive functioning in dementia (Acevedo & Loewenstein, 2007). For example, Spaced-Retrieval-Technique (SRT) in which the interval between the moment of presentation and the moment of retrieval is increased, makes it progressively more difficult for the patient to recall the information correctly. If the patient recalls the information incorrectly, the interval is shortened again. SRT appeals to implicit memory (Acevedo & Loewenstein, 2007). Implicit learning is also the basis for procedural motor learning, such as learning to dance, as well as for 'dual cognitive support' (Acevedo & Loewenstein, 2007). Dual cognitive support implies that by providing extra information during the encoding and the retrieval process, the person may be more able to organize the provided information. They also indicate that cognitive rehabilitation programs consisting of memory, communication, and problem-solving exercises are effective in dementia patients as well. In addition, training of ADL appears to be effective in Alzheimer's disease; the ADL improvements can be generalized to other untrained daily activities. Encouraging results concerning the effects of cognitive training on cognitive functioning in Alzheimer patients in particular also emerge from the review of Sitzer and co-workers (2006). For example, large effects (Cohen's d > .80) were observed concerning executive functions, and verbal and visual learning. However, larger effects were observed when the experimental group was compared to a placebo-free control group, instead of a control group that received a placebo. Another limitation is that this review only consisted of 6 randomized controlled trials. The authors conclude that cognitive training might have some beneficial effect in Alzheimer patients (Sitzer, Twamley, & Jeste, 2006).

6.3.8 Conclusions

The fact that in aging and even in dementia, the brain is able to use alternative strategies to complete a certain task, limits on one hand the use of neuropsychological tests to assess for example 'frontal' functions, by e.g., the Wisconsin Card Sorting Test. Elderly people will probably execute this task with more posterior situated brain areas than young people do. On the other hand, the presence of alternative neuronal functional circuits by which the elderly person functions at the highest possible level, may reduce the general feeling of 'therapeutic nihilism'. Particularly in dementia, this knowledge may be an invitation to further develop pharmacological and non-pharmacological interventions aimed at keeping these alternative circuits as active as possible, as long as possible.

6.4 Questions

1. Does bilateral brain activity during the performance of a task, support the 'compensation hypothesis'? Please explain.
2. Is bilateral brain activity characteristic for high-functioning older persons? Please explain.
3. What is the effect of aging on the prefrontal cortex during retrieval of information from memory store?
4. Could you give an example of intrahemispheric compensation in elderly people without dementia?
5. Are compensatory mechanisms also characteristic for cognitive functioning in Alzheimer's disease? Please explain.
6. Which hand motor functions can successfully be trained in aging?
7. Which aspect of hand motor function is not easy to train in older persons?
8. Please explain the phenomenon 'last in – first out'.
9. Why do Alzheimer patients walk with a larger sway during the course of the disease?
10. How could one decrease the larger sway observed in Alzheimer patients?
11. What are the clinical consequences of the 'last in – first out' phenomenon for the gait-related motor functions of the separate brain regions belonging to the SLF?
12. In a relatively early stage, frontotemporal dementia and vascular dementia are characterized by a loss of initiative. Does this have implications for the caring of these patients? Please explain.
13. Please explain why it might be worthwhile for patients in a relatively early stage of Alzheimer's disease to watch a video of other people walking?
14. Within the scope of the superior longitudinal fasciculus, which two brain areas play a role in the preparation of gait?
15. For which uncinate fasciculus-related area is the 'lat in – first out' phenomenon not applicable?
16. Why are patients with mild Huntington's disease still able to learn a graphomotor task by motor imagery?
17. Within the scope of the frontocerebellar connections, why is training 'gait speed' clinical important?
18. Within the scope of the frontostriatal connections, why is implicit, automatic motor learning still possible in Alzheimer's disease?
19. Within the scope of the cingulum, why is topographic orientation relatively spared in mild frontotemporal dementia and not in mild Alzheimer's disease?

20. Why should patients with mild to moderate Alzheimer's disease have the opportunity to explicitly practice over-learned motor activity such as walking? (think of intactness of specific brain areas).
21. Which subtype of dementia would show the most positive reaction to a rehabilitation program focused on gait?
22. In what way might cholinesterase inhibitors improve higher-level gait disturbances?
23. Which motor area seems to be involved in gait apraxia?
24. In Parkinson's disease, the effects of cholinesterase inhibitors on motor activity appear to be inconsistent. Please explain.
25. Which type of white matter is particularly vulnerable for cardiovascular risk factors?
26. Describe the cascade of events that starts with cardiovascular risk factors and finally results in dementia.
27. Describe the cascade of events that starts with insulin resistance and finally results in Alzheimer's disease.
28. Describe the cascade of events that starts with insulin resistance and finally results in type 2 diabetes mellitus.
29. Please explain the relationship between insulin and nitric oxide.
30. In which three components can an active lifestyle be subdivided?
31. Please explain how a rich social environment decreases the risk of death.
32. Please explain the relationship between level of education and Alzheimer's disease.
33. Please explain why exercise may lead to vasodilatation.
34. Is (an increase in) physical activity beneficial for the cognitive functioning of patients diagnosed with dementia?
35. Which three types of biological mechanisms underlie 'enriched environment'?
36. Is cognitive training effective in older persons without dementia and persons with Mild Cognitive Impairment (MCI)?
37. How effective is cognitive training in persons with dementia? Why should one consider the results of those studies with caution?

Chapter 7
Pain in dementia

7.1 Introduction

There is convincing evidence that the number of people above 65 years of age will increase substantially in the next decades and that age is the highest risk factor for dementia (Skoog, 2004). Since aging also coincides with a high rate of painful conditions, irrespective of the cognitive status (Horgas & Elliot, 2004), an increase in the number of demented patients with a painful condition can be anticipated. A striking finding from epidemiological and clinical studies is, however, that patients with dementia use fewer analgesics than non-demented elderly, underscoring undertreatment of pain in dementia (Herr & Decker, 2004). Undertreatment of pain in elderly persons with dementia could be caused by dementia-related problems in communication about pain, complicating pain assessment. The most frequently used instruments to assess pain in communicative and non-communicative patients will be discussed in this chapter. An important component that further contributes to the complexity of pain assessment in dementia is that pain experience may change by the neuropathology underlying the various subtypes of dementia, i. e., Alzheimer's disease, vascular dementia, and frontotemporal dementia (Scherder et al., 2003a). Results of the few available clinical studies examining pain in these subtypes of dementia are interpreted in relation with the dementia-related neuropathology in the medial and lateral pain systems, will be addressed in this chapter. Paucity in clinical and experimental pain studies is even more striking with respect to disorders with a high risk for cognitive impairment such as Parkinson's disease and multiple sclerosis. In these disorders, pain is a prominent clinical symptom in a stage in which the patients are cognitively intact. However, so far, no studies have examined possible changes in pain experience in a stage in which the patients become cognitively impaired. Of note is that the same problems concerning pain assessment and treatment holds for people with an intellectual disability, e.g., persons with Down syndrome, Prader-Willi, Williams syndrome. Similar to patients with dementia, it is hypothesized that the neuropathology in these disorders contributes to insight into possible changes in pain experience (de Knegt & Scherder, 2011).

It is concluded that a differentiation between the various subtypes of dementia and between various subtypes of persons with an intellectual disability, is essential to make progress in pain assessment and treatment.

7.2   (Under)treatment of pain in dementia

A lower use of analgesics, including non-steroidal anti-inflammatory drugs (NSAIDs), has frequently been observed in patients with dementia, compared to elderly persons without dementia (Hanlon et al., 1996; Schmader et al., 1998). One explanation might be that painful conditions like arthritis occur less frequently in persons with dementia (McCormick et al., 1994; Wolf-Klein et al., 1988). However, in several studies the prevalence of osteoarticular pathologies was similar in both the elderly with and without dementia and the use of NSAIDs was still considerably less in the former group (Lucca, Tettamanti, Forloni, & Spagnoli, 1994; Ferrell, Ferrell, & Rivera, 1995). In patients with comparable painful conditions, the use of analgesics showed even an inverse relationship with the course of the disease (Fisher-Morris & Gellatly, 1997). An explanation is that the more the disease progresses, the less the patients are able to communicate about their pain.

A low use of analgesics is not restricted to musculoskeletal disorders. Marzinski (1991) found that only 13% of Alzheimer patients with a painful condition, e.g., metastatic colon cancer, used analgesics. Others observed that the oldest of a large group of cancer patients used fewer analgesics (Bernabei et al., 1998); one of the independent predictors of this finding was low cognitive performance. These findings are the more worrying since the prevalence of cancer increases with age (Luciani & Balducci, 2004). In sum, the majority of the above-mentioned results points to undertreatment of pain and may implicitly indicate a lack of adequate pain assessment.

With respect to pain treatment, there is paucity in studies examining the effectiveness of pain treatment strategies in dementia. Results of a recent double-blind, double-dummy, placebo-controlled, crossover study show that the level of discomfort in severely demented patients with a painful condition did not decrease after administration of 2,600-mg/d dose of acetaminophen, administered either regularly or as needed (Buffum, Sands, Miaskowski, Brod, & Washburn, 2004). The most obvious conclusion is that this dose is too low. Alternatively, the observed discomfort might not be related to pain in this patient group (Buffum, Miaskowski, & Sands, 2004). These findings underscore the complexity of pain assessment in non-communicative patients and urge the need for reliable pain assessment instruments.

7.3   Pain assessment

Of note is that the selection of pain assessment instruments is primarily determined by the communicative capacities of the patient, instead of the pain aspect one wants to assess, e.g., motivational-affective aspects or intensity of pain. Self-report pain rating scales such as verbal rating scales, visual analogue scales, and numeric rating scales, are administered to patients who can still communicate about their pain. In non-communicative patients, observation of physical signs and autonomic responses are the most appropriate methods to assess pain.

7.3.1 Communicative patients

Verbal pain rating scales, visual analogue scales and numeric pain rating scales
In a few studies the psychometric properties of verbal pain rating scales, visual analogue scales, and numerical scales that are most frequently used were examined (Chibnall & Tait, 2001; Taylor & Herr, 2003; Closs, Barr, Briggs, Cash, & Seers, 2004; Herr, Spratt, Mobily, & Richardson, 2004). Two verbal pain rating scales are the Verbal Description Scale (VDS) (Herr et al., 2004) and the Verbal Rating Scale (VRS) (Melzack, 1975). The VDS is composed of adjectives that represent different levels of pain experience, ranging from 'no pain' to 'the most intense pain imaginable', and the VRS consists of labels describing the nature of pain, e.g., distressing. Others use the expression 'VRS' also for describing pain levels such as 'moderate' (Closs et al., 2004). Visual analogue scales include the Mechanical Visual Analogue Scale (MVAS) (McGrath et al., 1996) and the Faces Pain Scale (FPS) (Bieri, Reeve, Champion, Addicoat, & Ziegler, 1990). The MVAS is a kind of thermometer with a plastic pointer that one can slide to the top (dark red colour) for the worst possible pain and to the bottom (light pink colour) for no pain. The FPS consists of line drawings of 7 faces, i.e., one neutral face and six faces which express increasing feelings of pain. Two examples of numeric rating scales are the 'numeric rating scale' (NRS) (Taylor & Herr, 2003) and the 21-point Box scale (BS-21) (Jensen, Miller, & Fisher, 1998). The former scale is a 1-10 horizontal scale, sometimes combined with the words 'no pain' at one end and 'worst possible pain' at the other end of the scale (Taylor & Herr, 2003). The BS-21 consists of 21 boxes on a horizontal line ranging from 0 ('no pain') to 100 ('pain as bad as it could be'), with intervals of 5 points. At each interval one box is added, i.e., one box is located at number 5 and four boxes piled on each other are located at number 20, and so forth.

Taylor and Herr (2003) administered the FPS, the VDS/VRS, the NRS, and the MVAS to 'cognitively impaired African American older adults' (mean score of the Mini-Mental State Examination (MMSE): 20; range: 7-29). The authors indicate that all participants were able to rate their pain by means of all four scales, of which the FPS was the most preferred one. Similar scales were administered to cognitively impaired elderly (mean MMSE-score: 15; range: 10-17) who were primarily of Caucasian origin (Closs et al., 2004). The majority of these elderly persons were able to use the scales. The scale by which they could best describe the intensity of the pain was the VRS. In another study, the BS-21 appeared to be the best scale with respect to reliability and construct validity, in comparison with the VRS and FPS (Chibnall & Tait, 2001). Most of these scales are notated as 'intensity' scales (Taylor & Herr, 2003); the FPS and the VDS/VRS might also appeal to affective components of pain.

Taken together, the here reviewed studies indicate that all scales show quite acceptable and comparable psychometric properties; the preferred scale seems to be dependent on the ethnic background. Importantly, the studies described above reported that all or the majority of the cognitively impaired elderly were able to use the scales. Despite this encouraging outcome, additional assessment of cognitive functioning might be valuable. For example, Herr and co-workers (2004) administered the Cognitive Capacity Screening Examination (CCSE) (Jacobs, Bernhard, Delgado, & Strain, 1977) and a clock drawing test (Dastoor, Schwartz, & Kurzman, 1991) to control for abstract thinking, a prerequisite for an appropriate use of the MVAS.

7.3.2 Non-communicative patients

Observation scales

Pain assessment in non-communicative patients relies primarily on observation scales (Herr & Decker, 2004). Widely used observation scales are the Discomfort Scale-Dementia of Alzheimer type (DS-DAT) (Hurley, Volicer, Hanrahan, Houde, & Volicer, 1992), the Assessment of Discomfort in Dementia (ADD) (Kovach, Weissman, Griffie, Matson, & Muchka, 1999), the Pain Assessment in Advanced Dementia scale (PAINAD scale) (Warden, Hurley, & Volicer, 2003), the Checklist for Nonverbal Pain Indicators (CNPI) (Feldt, 2001), the Non-Communicative Patient's Pain Assessment Instrument (NOPPAIN) (Snow et al., 2004), and the Pain Assessment Checklist for Seniors with Limited Ability to Communicate (PAC-SLAC) (Fuchs-Lacelle & Hadjistavropoulos, 2004).

These scales consist of items that are focused on the intensity and location of pain, the affective components of pain, and autonomic responses to pain like breathing and sweating. Another communality of these scales is the assessment of the facial expression of pain. Facial actions can be coded by a specific system: the Facial Action Coding System (FACS) (Ekman & Friesen, 1978). The FACS appeared to reliably assess pain in older persons who underwent a knee replacement (Hadjistavropoulos, LaChapelle, Hadjistavropoulos, Green, & Asmundson, 2002). More specifically, the FACS not only assessed the presence/absence of pain but also the varying levels of pain related to the various degrees of activity (Hadjistavropoulos et al., 2002). In another recent study with patients with severe dementia, facial expressions before and during the caring of decubitus ulcers were video-taped. The 18 observers highly agreed on the presence/absence of pain but not on its intensity (Manfredi, Breuer, Meier, & Libow, 2003a).

A disadvantage of observation scales is the necessary assumption that signs which are normally indicative for pain are also representative for pain in the demented elderly (Kovach et al., 1999). This assumption is however doubtful (Herr & Decker, 2004). For example, 'absence of a relaxed body posture', one of the items of the DS-DAT, may also be the reflection of extrapyramidal symptoms that can occur in Alzheimer's disease (Caligiuri, Peavy, & Galasko, 2001). Extrapyramidal symptoms might also disturb the facial expression of pain in patients with Lewy body dementia (Aarsland, Ballard, McKeith, Perry, & Larsen, 2001). Interestingly, also in patients with a right-sided temporal lobe variant of frontotemporal dementia, a decrease in facial expression has been observed (Edwards-Lee et al., 1997). In other words, absence of a facial expression of pain is not evidence of absence of pain. This same conclusion will hold for measuring autonomic responses to pain that will be discussed in the next section.

7.3.3 Autonomic responses to pain

Only one clinical and two experimental studies have been performed in which autonomic responses of Alzheimer patients to pain were examined. Responses to venipuncture, as part of a physical examination, were examined in Alzheimer patients and elderly persons without dementia (Porter et al., 1996). In comparison with the latter group, Alzheimer patients were less able to anticipate the puncture, reflected in less heart rate increase. Consequently, due to a lack of preparation, heart rate increased more in demented patients than in non-demented elderly persons during the venipuncture itself. Rainero and co-workers (2000) applied a painful electrical stimulus at the wrist of Alzheimer patients. Alzheimer patients only showed a normal increase in systolic blood pressure if the intensity of the painful stimulus was high but showed no autonomic responses to a mild painful stimulus. It is of note that the increase in heart frequency did not follow the same pattern: after painful electrical stimulation with a high intensity the increase in heart frequency remained much lower in Alzheimer patients compared to elderly persons without dementia. In other words, in Alzheimer's disease subparts of the autonomic nervous system react differently to pain. In another study with Alzheimer patients, a negative correlation was observed between heart rate responses and degree of cognitive impairment, in the presence of normal tactile and pain threshold (Benedetti et al., 2004). This finding which implies that autonomic responses to pain deteriorate whereas the processing of tactile and painful stimuli is still possible, underscores that a lack of autonomic responses needs not to be representative for a lack of pain.

In sum, measuring autonomic responses appears not to be a reliable method to assess pain in Alzheimer's disease. However, experimental pain studies have not been performed in other subtypes of dementia which neuropathology may differently affect autonomic responses to pain and hence pain experience.

7.3.4 Pain in dementia and in disorders with a high risk for cognitive impairment; its relationship with the medial and lateral pain systems

Findings from experimental and clinical studies that have examined pain experience in various subtypes of dementia (Alzheimer's disease, vascular dementia, and frontotemporal dementia) and two disorders with a high risk for cognitive impairment, i.e., Parkinson's disease and multiple sclerosis will be presented in this paragraph. However, in order to relate these findings to the neuropathology in the medial and lateral pain systems, brain areas that belong to both systems and aspects of pain that are processed by both systems will be discussed first.

The medial and lateral pain systems
The anatomical complexity of the medial and lateral pain system is a reflection of the multi-faceted nature of pain. In this paragraph, the focus will be on those areas of the medial and lateral pain systems that constitute the main framework of both systems (see figure 1) and of which the majority is affected in one or more subtypes of dementia, Parkinson's disease and multiple sclerosis (see figures 2–6). For a comprehensive description of ascending pathways and connections between the areas that belong to the two pain systems, see Willis and Westlund (1997).

Medial pain system. Thalamic nuclei, among which medial and intralaminar nuclei, receive nociceptive information either directly through the spinothalamic tract (STT) or indirectly through the spinoreticular and spinomesencephalic tract (SRT and SMT, respectively). Subsequently, the thalamus transmits information to the anterior cingulate cortex (ACC), insula, parietal operculum (PO), and the secondary somatosensory cortex (SII). Areas of the reticular formation such as the locus coeruleus (LC) and parabrachial nucleus (PBN) convey nociceptive information to the amygdala, hippocampus and the hypothalamic nuclei among which the paraventricular nucleus (PVN) (Vogt & Sikes, 2000; Rüb et al., 2002; Sewards & Sewards, 2002). In the PVN, oxytocin and arginine-vasopressin are produced, the latter co-localized with corticotrophin-releasing hormone (CRH) (Raadsheer, Tilders, & Swaab, 1994; Ishunina & Swaab, 2002; Swaab, 2003). The tuberomammillary nucleus (TMN) is the only histaminergic nucleus of the brain (Raadsheer et al., 1994; Ishunina & Swaab, 2002; Swaab, 2003). Histamine, oxytocin, arginine-

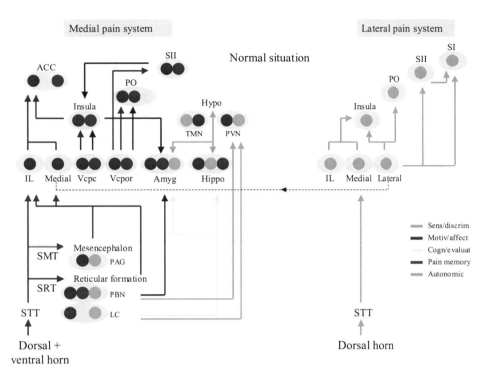

Figure 1. (Sub)cortical areas and pathways belonging to the medial and lateral pain system in a normal situation. Note that the majority of the presented brain areas contributes to more than one pain modality. STT: spinothalamic tract; SRT: spinoreticular tract; SMT: spinomesencephalic tract; LC: locus coeruleus; PBN: parabrachial nucleus; PAG: periaqueductal gray; IL: intralaminar thalamic nuclei; Medial: medial thalamic nuclei; Vcpc: ventral caudal parvocellular nucleus; Vcpor: ventral caudal portae nucleus; Amyg: amygdala; Hippo: hippocampus; Hypo: hypothalamus; TMN: tuberomamillary nucleus; PVN: paraventricular nucleus; PO: parietal operculum; ACC: anterior cingulate cortex; SII: secondary somatosensory area; SI: primary somatosensory area; ——— : contact between the medial and lateral pain system. Sens/discrim: sensory/discriminative aspects of pain; Motiv/affect: motivational/affective aspects of pain; Cogn/evaluat: cognitive/evaluative aspects of pain. Reprinted with permission from Scherder, E.J.A., Sergeant, J.A., & Swaab, D.F. (2003). Pain processing in dementia and its relation to neuropathology. Lancet Neurology, 2(11), 677-686. Lancet Ltd, London.

vasopressin and CRH are neuroactive compounds with an anti-nociceptive effect (Swaab et al., 2004).

With respect to the various aspects of pain, the medial pain system is involved in the motivational/affective aspects, cognitive/evaluative aspects, memory for pain, and autonomic aspects of pain (Vogt & Sikes, 2000; Sewards & Sewards, 2002).

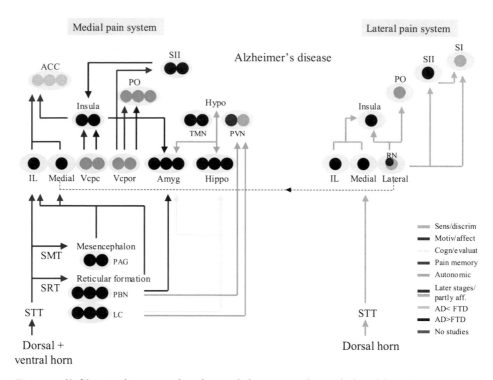

Figure 2. (Sub)cortical areas and pathways belonging to the medial and lateral pain system in Alzheimer's disease (AD). Note that the majority of the areas belonging to particularly the medial pain system are affected in AD. STT: spinothalamic tract; SRT: spinoreticular tract; SMT: spino-mesencephalic tract; LC: locus coeruleus; PBN: parabrachial nucleus; PAG: periaqueductal gray; IL: intralaminar thalamic nuclei; Medial: medial thalamic nuclei; Lateral: lateral thalamic nuclei; RN: reticular nucleus; Vcpc: ventral caudal parvocellular nucleus; Vcpor: ventral caudal portae nucleus; Amyg: amygdala; Hippo: hippocampus; Hypo: hypothalamus; TMN: tuberomamillary nucleus; PVN: paraventricular nucleus; PO: parietal operculum; ACC: anterior cingulate cortex; SII: secondary somatosensory area; SI: primary somatosensory area; —— : contact between the medial and lateral pain system. Sens/discrim: sensory/discriminative aspects of pain; Motiv/affect: motivational/affective aspects of pain; Cogn/evaluat: cognitive/evaluative aspects of pain; Later stages/partly affected: information about pathology exists only for the thalamic reticular nucleus which is affected in the later stages of AD (Braak ADFTD: more affected in AD than in FTD; A: amygdala; Hippo: hippocampus; LC: locus coeruleus. Reprinted with permission from Scherder, E.J.A., Sergeant, J.A., & Swaab, D.F. (2003), idem. Lancet Ltd, London.

Lateral pain system.

The STT also conveys information to the lateral thalamus which project to the insula, PO, SII, and the primary somatosensory cortex (SI). The lateral pain system plays a crucial role in the sensory/discriminative aspects of pain (Vogt & Sikes, 2000; Sewards & Sewards, 2002).

7.3.5 Clinical and experimental studies

Alzheimer's disease. By means of visual analogue scales among which the FPS (Bieri et al., 1990), pain was assessed in patients in a relatively early stage and mid-stage of Alzheimer's disease and in elderly persons without dementia (Scherder & Bouma, 2000). The number of painful conditions such as arthrosis/arthritis did not differ between the groups and with respect to the nature of the painful conditions, fractures occurred more frequently only in elderly in a more advanced stage. Elderly persons without dementia indicated to experience significantly more pain than patients with Alzheimer's disease, irrespective of its stage. It is of note that within the Alzheimer group, patients in a relatively early stage reported more pain than elderly persons in a more advanced stage of the disease. In a follow-up study similar pain assessment instruments were administered three times a day during two different periods, to reduce the influence of loss of memory for pain on patients' pain experience (Scherder et al., 2001).

The results were the same as in the previous study: Alzheimer patients reported to experience less pain than elderly persons without dementia. One of the flaws in these studies is that despite that the patient understands the concept of the scale it remains obscure if the patient is able to translate his own pain into the rating on the pain scales, truly a cognitive process.

The application of experimental pain stimuli demands less from cognitive functioning. Benedetti and co-workers (1999) applied electrical stimuli and ischemia of the arm and demonstrated that, compared to elderly persons without dementia, patients with Alzheimer's disease had the same pain threshold but a significant higher pain tolerance. This latter experimental outcome confirms the clinical outcome: Alzheimer patients may experience a decrease in the motivational/affective aspects of pain (Scherder et al., 2003a). In another experimental study it was observed that the increase in systolic blood pressure was similar in both Alzheimer patients and non-demented elderly persons only when the experimental pain stimulus had a high intensity (Rainero, Vighetti, Bergamasco, Pinessi, & Benedetti, 2000). In addition, an experimental pain stimulus of a low intensity induced heart rate increases that were smaller in Alzheimer patients than in elderly without dementia, suggesting a higher threshold for autonomic activation in Alzheimer's disease (Rainero et al., 2000).

The decrease in the motivational/affective aspects of pain in Alzheimer's disease is in agreement with the degeneration in the majority of the areas of the medial pain system (see figure 2). More specifically, the degeneration of the amygdala and hippocampus (Foundas, Leonard, Mahoney, Agee, & Heilman, 1997; Callen, Black, Gao, & Caldwell, 2002) might be responsible for a decline in memory for pain and, together with the TMN (Swaab, 1997), for the blunting of the autonomic responses. Furthermore, one could hypothesize that due to atrophy of the amygdala, hippocampus, LC, ACC and SII, cognitive/evaluative aspects of pain are deteriorated as well. Particularly in persistent pain, a type of pain that is most prevalent in elderly persons in a nursing home setting (Helme & Gibson, 2001), cognitive processes such as anticipation of the future and behavioural responses to pain, are most important (Price, 2000). As can be seen in figure 2, nociceptive information can still be transmitted to SI which might explain that the pain threshold (lateral pain system; sensory-discriminative aspects of pain) in Alzheimer's disease is not different from the pain threshold in elderly persons without dementia (Benedetti et al., 1999). The lateral pain system does show some functional decline in Alzheimer's disease though since, compared to elderly persons without dementia, the sensory threshold was elevated in Alzheimer's disease (Gibson, Voukelatos, Ames, Flicker, & Helme, 2001).

Vascular dementia. In only one study pain was assessed in patients with 'possible' vascular dementia (Scherder et al., 2003b). In that study the prevalence of osteoporosis was higher in the elderly persons without dementia while diabetes neuropathy occurred more frequently in elderly with vascular dementia. The scores on the scales that were also used in the above described Alzheimer's disease studies showed that elderly persons with vascular dementia indicated to suffer more from pain (motivational/affective aspects) than elderly persons without dementia.

An explanation for this finding is that white matter lesions, a neuropathological hallmark of vascular dementia (Barber et al., 1999), causes a disconnection between cortical areas and between cortical and subcortical areas (Mori, 2002), resulting in a so-called deafferentiation pain (Farrell, Katz, & Helme, 1996). For example, white matter lesions may disrupt connections between the intralaminar thalamic nuclei and SII (Schmahmann & Leifer, 1992) (see figure 3). This explanation could not be confirmed in the here described study, since brain imaging data were not available. A possible decline in the other four dimensions of pain will depend on where in the brain infarctions have occurred.

Frontotemporal dementia. In only one study so far the pain experience of patients with frontal variant frontotemporal dementia was assessed and compared to the pain experience of those with Alzheimer's disease and vascular dementia (Bathgate, Snowden, Varma, Blackshaw, & Neary, 2001). A remarkable finding was that in comparison with the latter two groups, elderly people with frontal variant frontotemporal dementia indicated to experience significantly less pain.

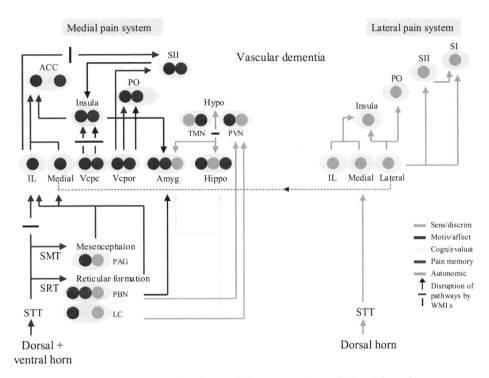

Figure 3. (Sub)cortical areas and pathways belonging to the medial and lateral pain system in Vascular dementia. Note the disconnections between the various brain areas. STT: spinothalamic tract; SRT: spinoreticular tract; SMT: spinomesencephalic tract; LC: locus coeruleus; PBN: parabrachial nucleus; PAG: periaqueductal gray; IL: intralaminar thalamic nuclei; Medial: medial thalamic nuclei; Vcpc: ventral caudal parvocellular nucleus; Vcpor: ventral caudal portae nucleus; Amyg: amygdala; Hippo: hippocampus; Hypo: hypothalamus; TMN: tuberomamillary nucleus; PVN: paraventricular nucleus; PO: parietal operculum; ACC: anterior cingulate cortex; SII: secondary somatosensory area; SI: primary somatosensory area; ——— : contact between the medial and lateral pain system. Sens/discrim: sensory/discriminative aspects of pain; Motiv/affect: motivational/affective aspects of pain; Cogn/evaluat: cognitive/evaluative aspects of pain; WMLs: white matter lesions. Reprinted with permission from Scherder, E.J.A., Sergeant, J.A., & Swaab, D.F. (2003), idem. Lancet Ltd, London.

Possibly the more severe metabolic decline in the frontal variant of frontotemporal dementia, as indicated by the stronger decrease in cerebral blood flow in the prefrontal cortex and anterior cingulate cortex, in comparison with e.g., Alzheimer's disease (see figure 3 and 4) (Varrone et al., 2002), could explain this finding, since these areas play an important role in the processing of motivational/affective aspects of pain. Although the amygdala and hippocampus are less affected in frontotemporal dementia than in Alzheimer's disease (figure 4) (Laakso et al., 2000; Boccardi et al., 2002), one should take a decline in the cognitive/evaluative aspects, the autonomic responses evoked by pain and the memory for pain into consideration when assessing pain in patients with frontotemporal dementia.

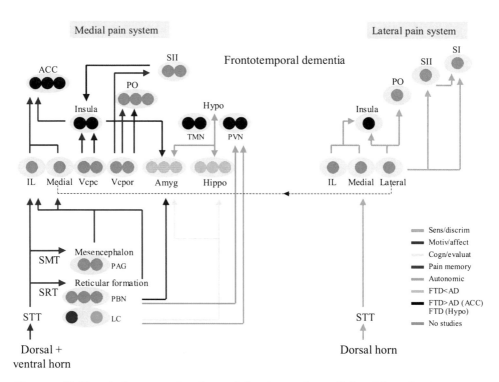

Figure 4. (Sub)cortical areas and pathways belonging to the medial and lateral pain system in frontotemporal dementia (FTD). Note that the prefrontal cortex which is more affected in FTD than in Alzheimer's disease (AD) (Varrone et al., 2002) is not indicated in the figure. STT: spinothalamic tract; SRT: spinoreticular tract; SMT: spinomesencephalic tract; LC: locus coeruleus; PBN: parabrachial nucleus; PAG: periaqueductal gray; IL: intralaminar thalamic nuclei; Medial: medial thalamic nuclei; Vcpc: ventral caudal parvocellular nucleus; Vcpor: ventral caudal portae nucleus; Amyg: amygdala; Hippo: hippocampus; Hypo: hypothalamus; TMN: tuberomamillary nucleus; PVN: paraventricular nucleus; PO: parietal operculum; ACC: anterior cingulate cortex; SII: secondary somatosensory area; SI: primary somatosensory area; —— : contact between the medial and lateral pain system. Sens/discrim: sensory/discriminative aspects of pain; Motiv/affect: motivational/affective aspects of pain; Cogn/evaluat: cognitive/evaluative aspects of pain; FTDAD: more affected in FTD than in AD; insu: insula. Reprinted with permission from Scherder, E.J.A., Sergeant, J.A., & Swaab, D.F. (2003), idem. Lancet Ltd, London.

7.3.6 Pain in Parkinson's disease and multiple sclerosis

Since a possible change in pain experience has not been examined in cognitively impaired patients with Parkinson's disease or multiple sclerosis, only studies in which pain was assessed in cognitively intact patients will be discussed.

Parkinson's disease. Pain was one of the dependent variables in several studies that focused on the influence of Parkinson's disease on the quality of life. In one study, a significant association between the progression of Parkinson's disease and an increase in pain was observed over a period of four years (Karlsen, Tandberg, Årsland, & Larsen, 2000). Importantly, the patients were not cognitively impaired (average Mini Mental-State Examination score after 4 years: 26.2). Similar findings were reported in another longitudinal study, in which pain was assessed over a three-year period (Schenkman, Wei Zhu, Cutson, & Whetten-Goldstein, 2001). In two reviews, a considerable number of somatic pain syndromes including musculoskeletal disorders such as limb rigidity, radicular-neuropathic disorders like restless legs syndrome, dystonia, akathisia, neck pain, and headache have been described in relation to Parkinson's disease (Waseem & Gwinn-Hardy, 2001; Ford, 1998). One non-somatically based pain syndrome with a less clear aetiology comprises primary sensory symptoms (Chudler & Dong, 1995) and is considered a type of 'central pain' (Schott, 1985; Ford, 1998; Waseem & Gwinn-Hardy, 2001).

Based on the location of the neuropathology, it is argued that Lewy bodies and Lewy neurites in areas such as the coeruleus-subcoeruleus region, the nucleus gigantocellularis and the bulbar nuclei, that normally inhibit nociceptive transmission at the spinal dorsal horn (Jones, 1991; Zhuo & Gebhart, 1991), are responsible for the clinically observed increase in motivational-affective aspects of pain (see figure 5). As can be seen in figure 5, also the other aspects of pain can still be processed.

Multiple sclerosis. Evidence of the presence of pain in multiple sclerosis emerges from various reviews of the most frequently occurring pain syndromes in multiple sclerosis. These pain syndromes include trigeminal neuralgia, somatic pain such as back pain and pain related to spasticity, visceral pain most frequently caused by spasms of the bladder, and a variety of other painful conditions like optic neuritis and an acute radicular syndrome (Moulin, 1989; Kerns, Kassirer, & Otis, 2002; Solaro, Lunardi, & Mancardi, 2003). In addition, dysaesthesia, a type of 'central pain' that consists of unpleasant sensations as a reaction to touch, has been described in patients with multiple sclerosis (Kerns et al., 2002; Bacher Svendsen et al., 2003; Solaro et al., 2003). Others confirmed the presence of central pain in multiple sclerosis (Nurmikko, 2000) which might also be reflected in the aetiology

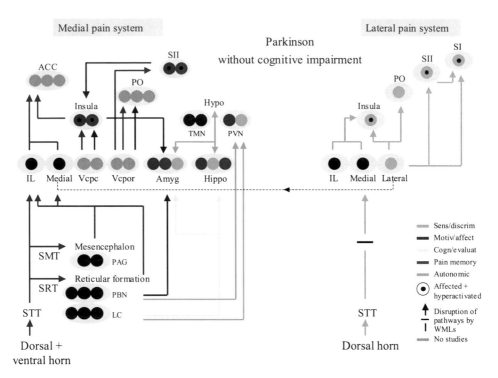

Figure 5. (Sub)cortical areas and pathways of the medial and lateral pain systems in Parkinson's disease without cognitive impairment. STT: spinothalamic tract; SRT: spinoreticular tract; SMT: spinomesencephalic tract; LC: locus coeruleus; PBN: parabrachial nucleus; PAG: periaqueductal gray; IL: intralaminar thalamic nuclei; Medial: medial thalamic nuclei; Lateral: lateral thalamic nuclei; RN: reticular nucleus; Vcpc: ventral caudal parvocellular nucleus; Vcpor: ventral caudal portae nucleus; Amyg: amygdala; Hippo: hippocampus; Hypo: hypothalamus; TMN: tuberoma-millary nucleus; PVN: paraventricular nucleus; PO: parietal operculum; ACC: anterior cingulate cortex; SII: secondary somato-sensory area; SI: primary somatosensory area; ——: contact be-tween the medial and lateral pain system. Sens/discrim: sensory/discriminative aspects of pain; Motiv/affect: motivational/ affective aspects of pain; Cogn/evaluat: cognitive/evaluative aspects of pain.

of severe acute headaches (Haas, Kent, & Friedman, 1993) and painful tonic sei-zures (Shibasaki & Kuroiwa, 1974). The results of a recent clinical study show that multiple sclerosis patients 1) experienced a higher pain intensity than a reference group; 2) needed more pain treatment (drugs, physiotherapy); and 3) experienced pain at more locations (Bacher Svendsen et al., 2003).

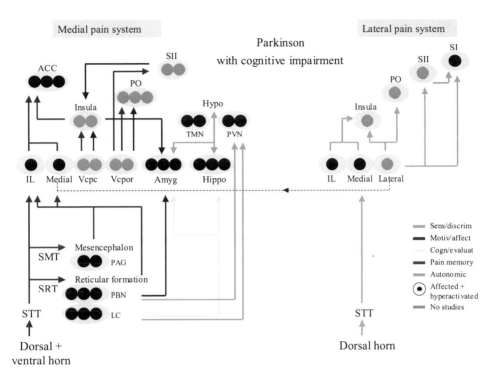

Figure 6. (Sub)cortical areas and pathways of the medial and lateral pain systems in Multiple Sclerosis (MS) without cognitive impairment. STT: spinothalamic tract; SRT: spinoreticular tract; SMT: spinomesencephalic tract; LC: locus coeruleus; PBN: parabrachial nucleus; PAG: periaqueductal gray; IL: intralaminar thalamic nuclei; Medial: medial thalamic nuclei; Lateral: lateral thalamic nuclei; RN: reticular nucleus; Vcpc: ventral caudal parvocellular nucleus; Vcpor: ventral caudal portae nucleus; Amyg: amygdala; Hippo: hippocampus; Hypo: hypothalamus; TMN: tuberomamillary nucleus; PVN: paraventricular nucleus; PO: parietal operculum; ACC: anterior cingulate cortex; SII: secondary somatosensory area; SI: primary somatosensory area; ——: contact between the medial and lateral pain system. Sens/discrim: sensory/discriminative aspects of pain; Motiv/affect: motivational/affective aspects of pain; Cogn/evaluat: cognitive/evaluative aspects of pain.

Similar to vascular dementia, white matter lesions are probably the cause of an increase in motivational-affective aspects of pain in multiple sclerosis, by disrupting cortical and subcortical-cortical connections (deafferentiation). Since areas of the medial pain system (e.g., insula) are affected but still show enhanced activation as a response to sensorimotor activity (Rocca et al., 2002), it is suggested that these areas are still able to process sensory information.

7.4 Summary

The low use of analgesics in elderly patients with dementia compared to elderly with a normal mental status strongly indicates undertreatment of pain in patients with dementia. Undertreatment of pain can only be prevented by the application of reliable pain assessment instruments. It is therefore most encouraging that the evaluation of psychometric properties of the most frequently used pain rating scales are the core issue in studies (Chibnall & Tait, 2001; Taylor & Herr, 2003; Herr et al., 2004; Closs et al., 2004). With respect to pain treatment, it is important to realize that most pain assessment instruments focus on just one aspect of pain. Verbal, visual, and numeric pain rating scales that are administered to communicative patients primarily measure quantitative aspects of pain such as the presence/ absence of pain and intensity (Taylor & Herr, 2003; Horgas & Elliott, 2004). Observation scales, developed for patients with severe cognitive decline (Herr & Decker, 2004), additionally assess qualitative aspects of pain like motivational-affective aspects. Since, besides pain intensity, also these latter aspects of pain require treatment (Sewards & Sewards, 2002), pain assessment should primarily focus on both aspects, irrespective of the patients' communicative abilities. In other words, observation scales should be applied to communicative patients as well. It should be noted, however, that the absence of e.g. facial expressions and autonomic responses does not imply that the patient is not in pain. These expressions of pain can be blurred by the neuropathology underlying the specific subtype of dementia. The fact that clinical studies have shown that the change in pain experience differs between the various subtypes of dementia (Scherder et al., 2003a) further stresses the importance of including the neuropathology, characteristic for each subtype of dementia (e.g., atrophy and white matter lesions) into pain assessment.

Taken together, the development of reliable pain assessment instruments together with insight into the neuropathology responsible for the patients' cognitive impairment will improve the detection of pain in dementia considerably.

Pain is a prominent clinical symptom in disorders such as Parkinson's disease and multiple sclerosis (Waseem & Gwinn-Hardy, 2001; Bacher Svendsen et al., 2003). Moreover, cognitive impairment occurs in later stages of Parkinson's disease and multiple sclerosis in a large number of patients, e.g., 40% in Parkinson's disease (Emre, 2003) and 65% in multiple sclerosis (Halper et al., 2003) and its influence on pain experience has not been addressed so far.

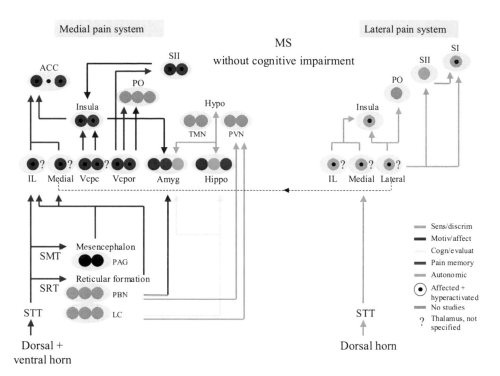

Figure 7. (Sub)cortical areas and pathways of the medial and lateral pain systems in Parkinson's disease with cognitive impairment. STT: spinothalamic tract; SRT: spinoreticular tract; SMT: spinomes-encephalic tract; LC: locus coeruleus; PBN: parabrachial nucleus; PAG: periaqueductal gray; IL: intralaminar thalamic nuclei; Medial: medial thalamic nuclei; Lateral: lateral thalamic nuclei; RN: reticular nucleus; Vcpc: ventral caudal parvocellular nucleus; Vcpor: ventral caudal portae nucleus; Amyg: amygdala; Hippo: hippo-campus; Hypo: hypothalamus; TMN: tuberoma-millary nucleus; PVN: paraventricular nucleus; PO: parietal operculum; ACC: anterior cingulate cortex; SII: secondary somatosensory area; SI: primary somato-sensory area; ——: contact between the medial and lateral pain system. Sens/discrim: sensory/ discriminative aspects of pain; Motiv/affect: motivational/affective aspects of pain; Cogn/evaluat: cognitive/evaluative aspects of pain.

Based on the neuropathology that coincides with cognitive impairment and affect areas of the medial and lateral pain systems, one could generate interesting hypotheses about possible changes in pain in both disorders. For example, due to Lewy bodies and Lewy neurites in the anterior cingulated corte, the amygdala and the prefrontal cortex in the cognitively impaired stage of Parkinson's disease (Jellinger, 2003), one could anticipate a decrease in motivational-affective aspects, cognitive-evaluative aspects, autonomic responses to pain, and memory of pain.

With respect to multiple sclerosis, a progressive increase in white matter lesions in a stage in which patients become cognitively impaired (Sperling et al.,

2001) may further enhance the suffering from motivational-affective aspects of pain.

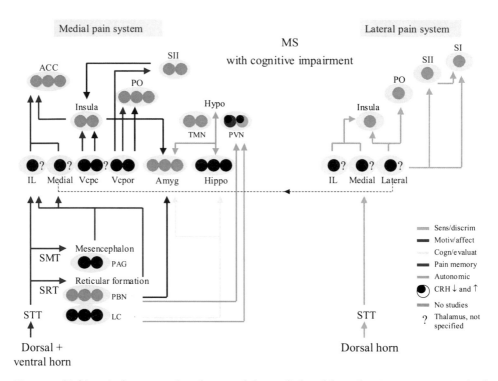

Figure 8. (Sub)cortical areas and pathways of the medial and lateral pain systems in Multiple Sclerosis (MS) with cognitive impairment. STT: spinothalamic tract; SRT: spinoreticular tract; SMT: spinomesencephalic tract; LC: locus coeruleus; PBN: parabrachial nucleus; PAG: periaqueductal gray; IL: intralaminar thalamic nuclei; Medial: medial thalamic nuclei; Lateral: lateral thalamic nuclei; RN: reticular nucleus; Vcpc: ventral caudal parvocellular nucleus; Vcpor: ventral caudal portae nucleus; Amyg: amygdala; Hippo: hippocampus; Hypo: hypothalamus; TMN: tuberomamillary nucleus; PVN: paraven-tricular nucleus; PO: parietal operculum; ACC: anterior cingulate cortex; SII: secondary somatosensory area; SI: primary somatosensory area; ——: contact between the medial and lateral pain system. Sens/discrim: sensory/discriminative aspects of pain; Motiv/affect: motivational/affective aspects of pain; Cogn/evaluat: cognitive/evaluative aspects of pain.

There is no doubt that clinical and experimental pain studies on the influence of the various subtypes of dementia on pain are desperately needed; studies on disorders such as Parkinson's disease and multiple sclerosis during which course patients may become cognitively impaired should be a permanent part of this research.

7.4.1 Pain may cause agitation in dementia

One of the pain suppressing systems originates from the prefrontal cortex. Consequently, frontal lesions in dementia may cause an increase in pain experience. In addition, disinhibited impulse aggression may result from lesions of the ventromedial and orbitofrontal prefrontal cortex (Brower & Price, 2001; Siever, 2008; Witte et al., 2009). Support for such a process emerges from neuroimaging studies, using for example Positron Emission Tomography (PET), that show a relationship between aggression and prefrontal cortex dysfunction, i.e., anterior frontal, orbitofrontal, and ventromedial areas (Brower & Price, 2001; Seo & Patrick, 2008). Lesions of the ventromedial and orbitofrontal cortex causing disinhibition, and consequently, agitation/aggression, may occur in neurodegenerative disorders such as dementia (Siever, 2008). This issue will be addressed first. Subsequently, considering the role of the prefrontal cortex in pain suppression, I will highlight that prefrontal cortex lesions in dementia may not only cause agitation/aggression, but may also contribute to an increase in pain experience. Consequently, in dementia agitation/aggression could be related to pain.

Disinhibition, agitation, and the prefrontal cortex
A relationship between behavioral disinhibition and an increase in serotonin turnover in the prefrontal cortex has been observed in a transgenic mouse model of Alzheimer's disease (Adriani et al., 2006). Agitated/aggressive patients with dementia, in particular those suffering from Alzheimer's disease, showed neuropathology, i.e., hypoperfusion, reduced metabolism, atrophy, and cholinergic dysfunction in the dorsolateral prefrontal cortex, anterior cingulate cortex, and anterior temporal lobe (Sultzer et al. 1995; Cummings & Back, 1998; Hirono, Mega, Dinov, Mishkin, & Cummings, 2000; Bruen, McGeown, Shanks, & Venneri, 2008). An association between a decreased volume in the ventromedial prefrontal cortex and disinhibition has been confirmed in dementia, irrespective of its subtype (Rosen et al., 2005). In the behavioral variant of frontotemporal dementia, disinhibition is related to atrophy of the dorsolateral prefrontal and orbitofrontal cortex (Krueger et al., 2009; Massimo et al., 2009).

Pain suppression and the prefrontal cortex
In humans, a top-down inhibitory influence of the prefrontal cortex on ascending pain-transmitting pathways has been observed. For example, in healthy adults who received a heat stimulus at the forearm, results from Positron Emission Tomography show a negative correlation between activity in the dorsolateral prefrontal cortex and activity in the connection between the midbrain, medial thalamus and cingulate, an ascending connection that mediates nociceptive information to the

brain (Lorenz, Minoshima, & Casey, 2003; Casey, Lorenz, & Minoshima, 2003). Similar findings have been reported for cold-evoked pain (Mohr et al., 2008). Such a top-down process is further supported by a study with healthy adults in which Transcranial Magnetic Stimulation applied to the left prefrontal cortex caused an increase in thermal pain threshold (Borckhardt et al., 2007).

Relationship between agitation and pain in dementia

Studies addressed so far, clearly indicate that lesions of the prefrontal cortex may cause agitation and pain in patients with dementia. The question arises whether these two symptoms indeed co-occur in dementia and whether a causal relationship exists between the presence of pain and agitation, i.e., does an increase in pain provoke agitation in patients with dementia.

Indeed, in one study, a significant proportion of the variance in discomfort of patients with moderate to severe dementia (14%) was explained by agitation (Buffum et al., 2001). In other words, the presence of a painful condition may contribute to agitation in patients with dementia (Buffum et al., 2001). The relationship between agitation and pain has also been observed in older patients visiting a day care centre (Cohen-Mansfield & Werner, 1999). In that study, pain was a significant predictor of verbally non-aggressive agitation. In patients with dementia who received end-of-life care in a hospice, less complaints of pain coincided with less prevalence of restlessness, sleep problems, agitation, and aggressiveness, compared to those who were not enrolled in a hospice (Bekelman, Black, Shore, Kasper, & Rabins, 2005).

The question arises whether pain really causes agitation in dementia. Evidence for a causal relationship emerges from a study applying an opioid to patients with dementia (Manfredi et al., 2003b). In that study, a long-acting opioid (oxycodone, 10 mg every 12 hours, or 20 mg morphine a day for those with problems in swallowing pills), administered during 4 weeks, reduced the level of agitation only in the oldest patients (i.e., 85 years of age) who were in an advanced stage of dementia.

7.4.2 Pain in persons with an intellectual disability

Similar to patients with dementia, is the assessment and treatment of pain very complex in persons with an intellectual disability. Clinical studies on pain in this population are scarce; only epidemiological and experimental studies are available (for a review, see de Knegt & Scherder, 2011).

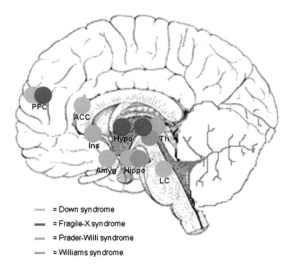

Figure 9. Pain-related grey matter neuropathology in the most prevalent subtypes of Intellectual Disability (ID): Down syndrome, Fragile-X syndrome, Prader-Willi syndrome, and Williams syndrome. PFC: prefrontal cortex; ACC: anterior cingulate cortex; Ins: insula; Hypo: hypothalamus; Th: thalamus; Amyg: amygdala; Hippo: hippocampus; LC: locus coeruleus. Reprinted with permission from de Knegt, N., & Scherder, E.J.A. (2011). Pain in adults with intellectual disabilities. Pain, 152(5), 971-974. Elsevier Science, Amsterdam.

Epidemiological studies show that persons with an intellectual disability suffer from musculoskeletal disorders. More specifically, adults with fragile-X syndrome suffer from excessive laxity of joints and scoliosis, whereas instability of the cervical spine is more characteristic for adults with cerebral palsy and persons with Down syndrome. This latter group may also suffer from a hip instability and osteoporosis (de Knegt & Scherder, 2011).

Results from experimental studies suggest that in reaction to an administered cold stimulus, verbal expressions of pain or discomfort are delayed and less precise in people with Down syndrome, compared to people in the control group. When receiving a hot stimulus, verbal expressions of pain or discomfort of persons with Down syndrome occur later than those without Down syndrome, and at a lower temperature (de Knegt & Scherder, 2011).

The review of de Knegt and Scherder (2011) further describes the neuropathology of the most prevalent subtypes of intellectual disabilities, in relation to pain experience (see figure 9). One of the hypotheses is that for example in persons with Down syndrome pain experience may on the one hand decrease due to degeneration of among others the hippocampus, amygdala, and insula whereas, on the other hand, pain experience may increase due to the degeneration of the prefrontal cortex and white matter.

One of the main conclusions of the review of de Knegt and Scherder (2011) is that in most subtypes of intellectual disability, the presence of musculoskeletal disorders has not been examined in relation to the experience of clinical pain. In other words, clinical pain studies with persons with intellectual disability are lacking.

7.5 Questions

1. Could you explain why the number of older persons with dementia suffering from pain will increase in the next decades?
2. Could you give some examples of an undertreatment of pain in dementia?
3. In general, on which grounds does one select the pain assessment instrument? Do you agree?
4. Please provide some examples of self-report pain rating scales.
5. Does people's ethnic background play a role in the selection of pain instruments?
6. Which aspects of pain are assessed by pain observation scales?
7. Please mention a major disadvantage of pain observation scales.
8. Please explain the influence of Alzheimer's disease on the autonomic responses to pain (in particular the studies of Rainero et al., 2000 and Benedetti et al., 2004).
9. In which aspects of pain is the medial pain system involved?
10. In which aspects of pain is the lateral pain system involved?
11. What is the influence of Alzheimer's disease on pain experience?
12. Is the pain experience in Alzheimer's disease stage-dependent?
13. What is the influence of Alzheimer's disease on pain threshold and pain tolerance? (Benedetti et al., 1999).
14. Could you explain the findings of Benedetti et al. (1999) with respect to the medial and lateral pain system?
15. Which brain areas might be responsible for a decrease in memory for pain in Alzheimer's disease?
16. Are patients with Alzheimer's disease still able to anticipate on the future and behavioural responses of pain? Which brain areas are involved?
17. Is the lateral pain system unaffected in Alzheimer's disease?
18. Please explain in terms of neuropathology the relationship between the motivational-affective aspects of pain and vascular dementia.
19. Compared to Alzheimer's disease, what is the influence of the frontal variant of frontotemporal dementia on pain? Could you explain this difference in terms of localization of neuropathology?
20. Could you explain why patients with Parkinson's disease without cognitive impairment suffer more from the motivational-affective aspects of pain?
21. What is meant by 'central pain'?
22. Do patients with multiple sclerosis experience more pain than people without multiple sclerosis? Please explain?
23. Is pain a prominent clinical symptom in Alzheimer's disease?
24. What is meant by 'deafferentiation' with respect to pain?

25. Why should pain observation scales also be applied to communicative patients?
26. What will happen to the experience of the various aspects of pain in Parkinson patients when cognitive function declines?
27. Why is an increase in suffering from pain in patients with multiple sclerosis who become cognitively impaired realistic?

Bibliography

Aalten, P., de Vugt, M.E., Lousberg, R., Korten, E., Jaspers, N., Senden, B., … Verhey, F.R.J. (2003). Behavioral problems in dementia: A factor analysis of the neuropsychiatric inventory. *Dementia and Geriatric Cognitive Disorders, 15*(2), 99-105.

Aarsland, D., Ballard, C., McKeith, I., Perry, R.H., & Larsen, J.P. (2001). Comparison of extrapyramidal signs in dementia with Lewy bodies and Parkinson's disease. *Journal of Neuropsychiatry and Clinical Neurosciences, 13*(3), 374-379.

Aarsland, D., Mosimann, U.P., & McKeith, I.G. (2004). Role of cholinesterase inhibitors in Parkinson's disease and dementia with Lewy bodies. *Journal of Geriatric Psychiatry and Neurology, 17*(3), 164-171.

Acevedo A., & Loewenstein, D.A. (2007). Nonpharmacological Cognitive Interventions in Aging and Dementia. *Journal of Geriatric Psychiatry and Neurology, 20*(4), 239-249.

Ackl, N., Ising, M., Schreiber, Y.A., Atiya, M., Sonntag, A., & Auer, D.P. (2005). Hippocampal metabolic abnormalities in mild cognitive impairment and Alzheimer's disease. *Neuroscience Letters, 384*(1-2), 23-28.

Adriani, W., Ognibene, E., Heuland, E., Ghirardi, O., Caprioli, A., & Laviola, G. (2006). Motor impulsivity in APP-SWE mice: A model of Alzheimer's disease. *Behavioural Pharmacology, 17*(5-6), 525-533.

Aggarwal, N.T., Wilson, R.S., Beck, T.L., Bienias, J.L., & Bennett, D.A. (2006). Motor dysfunction in mild cognitive impairment and the risk of incident Alzheimer's Disease. *Archives of Neurology, 63*(12), 1763-1769.

Alessi, C.A., & Schnelle, J.F. (2000). Approach to sleep disorders in the nursing home setting. *Sleep Medicine Reviews, 4*(1), 45-56.

Alexander, N.B., Mollo, J.M., Giordani, B., Ashton-Miller, J.A., Schultz, A.B., Grunawalt, J.A., & Foster, N.L. (1995). Maintenance of balance, gait patterns, and obstacle clearance in Alzheimer's disease. *Neurology, 45*(5), 908-914.

Almkwist, O., & Winblad, B. (1999). Early diagnosis of Alzheimer dementia based on clinical and biological factors. *European Archives of Psychiatry and Clinical Neuroscience, 249*(Suppl. 3), 3-9.

Andersen, B.B., Gundersen, H.J., & Pakkenberg, B. (2003). Aging of the human cerebellum: A stereological study. *The Journal of Comparative Neurology, 466*(3), 356-365.

Andin, U., Gustafson, L., Passant, U., & Brun, A. (2005). A clinico-pathological study of heart and brain lesions in vascular dementia. *Dementia and Geriatric Cognitive Disorders, 19*(4), 222-228.

Angevaren, M., Aufdemkampe, G., Verhaar, H.J.J., Aleman, A., & Vanhees, L. (2008). Physical activity and enhanced fitness to improve cognitive function in older people without known cognitive impairment. *Cochrane Database of Systematic Reviews, 3*, CD005381.

Anstey, K.J., Lord, S.R., & Williams, P. (1997). Strength in the lower limbs, visual contrast sensitivity, and simple reaction time predict cognition in older women. *Psychology and Aging, 12*(1), 137-144.

Ard, J.D., Grambow, S.C., Liu, D., Slentz, C.A., Kraus, W.E., & Svetkey, L.P. (2004). The effect of PREMIER interventions on insulin sensitivity. *Diabetes Care, 27*(2), 340-347.

Aron, A.R., Robbins, T.W., & Poldrack, R.A. (2004). Inhibition and the right inferior frontal cortex. *Trends in Cognitive Sciences, 8*(4),170-177.

Arriagada, P.V., Marzloff, K., & Hyman, B.T. (1992). Distribution of Alzheimer-type pathologic changes in nondemented elderly individuals matches the pattern in Alzheimer's disease. *Neurology, 42*(9), 1681-1688.

Ashford, D., Davids, K., & Bennett, S.J. (2007). Developmental effects influencing observational modelling: A meta-analysis. *Journal of Sports Science, 25*(5), 547-558.

Assaiante, C., & Amblard, B. (1993). Ontogenesis of head stabilization in space during locomotion in children: Influence of visual cues. *Experimental Brain Research, 93*(3), 499-515.

Babiloni, C., Babiloni, F., Carducci, F., Cincotti, F., Del Percio, C., De Pino, G., ... Rossini, P.M. (2000). Movement-related electroencephalographic reactivity in Alzheimer disease. *NeuroImage, 12*(2), 139-146.

Babiloni, C., Frisoni, G.B., Pievani, M., Vecchio, F., Infarinato, F., Geroldi, C., ... Rossini, P.M. (2007). White matter vascular lesions are related to parietal-to-frontal coupling of EEG rhythms in mild cognitive impairment. *Human Brain Mapping, 29*(12), 1355-1367.

Bäckman, L., & Farde, L. (2001). Dopamine and cognitive functioning: Brain imaging findings in Huntington's disease and normal aging. *Scandinavian Journal of Psychology, 42*(3), 287-296.

Bäckman, L., Jones, S., Berker, A.-K., Laukka, E.J., & Small, B.J. (2004). Multiple cognitive deficits during the transition to Alzheimer's disease. *Journal of Internal Medicine, 256*(3), 195-204.

Baddeley, A.D., & Wilson, B. (1988). Frontal amnesia and the dysexecutive syndrome. *Brain and Cognition, 7(2)*, 212-230.

Bakker, M., De Lange, F.P., Helmich, R.C., Scheeringa, R., Bloem, B.R., & Toni, I. (2008). Cerebral correlates of motor imagery of normal and precision gait. *NeuroImage, 41*(3), 998-1010.

Baltes, P.B., & Lindenberger, U. (1997). Emergence of a powerful connection between sensory and cognitive functions across the adult life span: A new window to the study of cognitive aging? *Psychology and Aging, 12*(1), 12-21.

Barber, R., Scheltens, P., Gholkar, A., Ballard, C., MvKeith, I., Ince, P., ... O'Brien, J. (1999). White matter lesions on magnetic resonance imaging in dementia with Lewy bodies, Alzheimer's disease, vascular dementia, and normal aging. *Journal of Neurology, Neurosurgery and Psychiatry, 67* (1), 66-72.

Barnden, L.R., Behin-Ain, S., Kwiatek, R., Casse, R., & Yelland, L. (2005). Age related preservation and loss in optimized brain SPECT. *Nuclear Medicine Communications, 26*(6), 497-503.

Barnes, J., Godbolt, A.K., Frost, C., Boyes, R.G., Jones, B.F., Scahill, R.I., ... Fox, N.C. (2007). Atrophy rates of the cingulate gyrus and hippocampus in Alzheimer's disease and FTLD. *Neurobiology of Aging, 28*(1), 20-28.

Barraclough, N.E., Xiao, D., Oram, M.W., & Perrett, D.I. (2006). The sensitivity of primate STS neurons to walking sequences and to the degree of articulation in static images. *Progress in Brain Research, 154*, 135-148.

Bartels, A.L., & Leenders, K.L. (2008). Brain imaging in patients with freezing of gait. *Movement Disorders, 23*(Suppl. 2), S461-S467.

Bathgate, D., Snowden, J.S., Varma, A., Blackshaw, A., & Neary, D. (2001). Behaviour in frontotemporal dementia, Alzheimer's disease and vascular dementia. *Acta Neurologica Scandinavica, 103* (6), 367-378.

Beauchet, O., Allali, G., Annweiler, C., Bridenbaugh, S., Assal, F., Kressig, R.W., & Herrmann, F.R. (2009). Gait variability among healthy adults: Low and high stride-to-stride variability are both a reflection of gait stability. *Gerontology, 55*(6), 702-706.

Becker, J.T., Davis, S.W., Hayashi, K.M., Meltzer, C.C., Toga, A.W., Lopez, O.L., & Thompson, P.M. (2006). Three-dimensional patterns of hippocampal atrophy in Mild Cognitive Impairment. *Archives of Neurology, 63*(1), 97-101.

Bekelman, D.B., Black, B.S., Shore, A.D., Kasper, J.D., & Rabins, P.V. (2005). Hospice Care in a cohort of elders with dementia and mild cognitive impairment. *Journal of Pain and Symptom Management, 30*(3), 208-214.

Bellgrove, M.A., Phillips, J.G., Bradshaw, J.L., Hall, K.A., Presnell, I., & Hecht, H. (1997). Response programming in dementia of the Alzheimer type: A kinematic analysis. *Neuropsychologia, 35*(3), 229-240.

Benedetti, F., Arduino, C., Vighetti, S., Asteggiano, G., Tarenzi, L., & Rainero, I. (2004). Pain reactivity in Alzheimer patients with different degrees of cognitive impairment and brain electrical activity deterioration. *Pain, 111*(1 2), 22 29.

Benedetti, F., Vighetti, S., Ricco, C., Lagna, E., Bergamasco, B., Pinessi, L., & Rainero, L. (1999). Pain threshold and pain tolerance in Alzheimer's disease. *Pain, 80*(1-2), 377-382.

Bernabei, R., Gambassi, G., Lapane, K., Landi, F., Gatsoni, C., Dunlop, R., ... Mor, V. (1998). Management of pain in elderly patients with cancer. *Journal of the American Medical Association, 279* (23), 1877-1882.

Bieri, D., Reeve, R.A., Champion, G.D., Addicoat, L., & Ziegler, J.B. (1990). The Faces Pain Scale for the self-assessment of the severity of pain experienced by children: Development, initial validation, and preliminary investigation for ratio scale properties. *Pain, 41*(2), 139-150.

Binkofski, F., & Buccino, G. (2006). The role of ventral premotor cortex in action execution and action understanding. *Journal of Physiology Paris, 99*(4-6), 396-405.

Black, J.E., Isaacs, K.R., & Greenough, W.T. (1991). Useful vs. successful aging: Some notes on experiential factors. *Neurobiology of Aging, 12*(4), 325-328.

Blankevoort, C.G., van Heuvelen, M.J.G., Boersma, F., Luning, H., de Jong, J., & Scherder, E.J.A. (2010). Review of effects of physical activity on strength, balance, mobility and ADL performance in elderly subjects with dementia. *Dementia and Geriatric Cognitive Disorders, 30*(5), 392-402.

Blass, J.P. (1993). Pathophysiology of the Alzheimer's syndrome. *Neurology, 43*(8) (suppl. 4), S25-S38.

Blesa, R., Mohr, E., Miletich, R.S., Hildebrand, K., Sampson, M., & Chase, T.N. (1996). Cerebral metabolic changes in Alzheimer's disease: Neurobehavioral patterns. *Dementia, 7*(5), 239-245.

Bobillier, P., Seguin, S., Petitjean, F., Salvert, D., Touret, M., & Jouvet, M. (1976). The raphe nuclei of the cat brain stem: A topographical atlas of their efferent projections as revealed by autoradiography. *Brain Research, 113*(3), 449-486.

Boccardi, M., Pennanen, C., Laakso, M.P., Testa, C., Geroldi, C., Soininen, I.I., & Frisoni, G.B. (2002). Amygdaloid atrophy in frontotemporal dementia and Alzheimer's disease. *Neuroscience Letters, 335*(2), 139-143.

Booth, J.R., Burman, D.D., Meyer, J.R., Lei, Z., Trommer, B.L., Davenport, N.D., ... Mesulam, M.M. (2003). Neural development of selective attention and response inhibition. *NeuroImage, 20*(2), 737-751.

Borckardt, J.J., Smith, A.R., Reeves, S.T., Weinstein, M., Kozel, F.A., Nahas, Z., ... George, M.S. (2007). Fifteen minutes of left prefrontal repetitive transcranial magnetic stimulation acutely increases thermal pain thresholds in healthy adults. *Pain Research & Management, 12*(4), 287-290.

Borroni, B., Alberici, A., Premi, E., Archetti, S., Garibotto, V., Agosti, C., ... Padovani, A. (2008). Brain magnetic resonance imaging structural changes in a pedigree of asymptomatic progranulin mutation carriers. *Rejuvenation Research, 11*(3), 585-595.

Borroni, B., Brambati, S.M., Agosti, C., Gipponi, S., Bellelli, G., Gasparotti, R., ... Padovani, A. (2007). Evidence of white matter changes on diffusion tensor imaging in frontotemporal dementia. *Archives of Neurology, 64*(2), 246-251.

Borroni, B., Perani, D., Archetti, S., Agosti, C., Paghera, B., Bellelli, G., ... Padovani, A. (2006). Functional correlates of Apolipoprotein E genotype in Frontotemporal Lobar Degeneration. *BMC Neurology, 6*, 31.

Bowler, J.V. (2002). The concept of vascular cognitive impairment. *Journal of the Neurological Sciences, 203*, 11-15.

Boyle, P.A., Cohen, R.A., Paul, R., Moser, D., & Gordon, N. (2002). Cognitive and motor impairments predict functional declines in patients with vascular dementia. *International Journal of Geriatric Psychiatry, 17*(2), 164-169.

Bozeat, S., Gregory, C.A., Ralph, M.A.L., & Hodges, J.R. (2000). Which neuropsychiatric and behavioural features distinguish frontal and temporal variants of frontotemporal dementia from Alzheimer's disease? *Journal of Neurology, Neurosurgery & Psychiatry, 69*(2), 178-186.

Braak, H., & Braak, E. (1991). Neuropathological staging of Alzheimer-related changes. *Acta Neuropathologica, 82*(4), 239-259.

Braver, T.S., & Barck, D.M. (2002). A theory of cognitive control, aging cognition, and neuromodulation. *Neuroscience and Biobehavioral Reviews, 26*(7), 809-817.

Brody, H. (1992). The aging brain. *Acta Neurologica Scandinavica, 137*(Suppl. 137), 40-44.

Brower, M.C., & Price, B.H. (2001). Neuropsychiatry of frontal lobe dysfunction in violent and criminal behaviour: A critical review. *Journal of Neurology, Neurosurgery and Psychiatry, 71*(6), 720-726.

Brown, L.A., Shumway-Cook, A., & Woollacott, M.H. (1999). Attentional demands and postural recovery: The effects of aging. *Journals of Gerontology Series A-Biological Sciences and Medical Sciences, 54*(4), M165–M171.

Brown, S., Martinez, M.J., & Parsons, L.M. (2006). The neural basis of human dance. *Cerebral Cortex, 16*(8), 1157-1167.

Bruen, P.D., McGeown, W.J., Shanks, M.F., & Venneri, A. (2008). Neuroanatomical correlates of neuropsychiatric symptoms in Alzheimer's disease. *Brain, 131*, 2455-2463.

Buckner, R.L. (2004). Memory and executive function in aging and AD: Multiple factors that cause decline and reserve factors that compensate. *Neuron, 44*(1), 195-208.

Buffum, M.D., Miaskowski, C., & Sands, L. (2001). A pilot study of the relationship between discomfort and agitation in patients with dementia. *Geriatric Nursing, 22*(2), 80-85.

Buffum, M.D., Sands, L., Miaskowski, C., Brod, M., & Washburn, A. (2004). A clinical trial of the effectiveness of regularly scheduled versus as-needed administration of acetaminophen in the management of discomfort in older adults with dementia. *Journal of the American Geriatrics Society, 52*(7), 1093-1097.

Bullock-Saxton, J.E., Wong, W.J., & Hogan, N.(2001). The influence of age on weight-bearing joint reposition sense of the knee. *Experimental Brain Research, 136*(3), 400-406.

Bürgel, U., Amunts, K., Hoemke, L., Mohlberg, H., Gilsbach, J.M., & Zilles, K. (2006). White matter fiber tracts of the human brain: Three-dimensional mapping at microscopic resolution, topography and intersubject variability. *NeuroImage, 29*(4), 1092–1105.

Burke, D.M., & MacKay, D.G. (1997). Memory, language, and aging. *Philosophical Transaction of the Royal Society of London, 352*(1363), 1845-1856.

Burton, E.J., McKeith, I.G., Burn, D.J., Williams, E.D., & O'Brien, J.T. (2004). Cerebral atrophy in Parkinson's disease with and without dementia: A comparison with Alzheimer's disease, dementia with Lewy bodies and controls. *Brain, 127*, 791-800.

Cabeza, R. (2002). Hemispheric asymmetry reduction in older adults: The HAROLD Model. *Psychology and Aging, 17*(1), 85-100.

Cabeza, R., Anderson, N.D., Locantore, J.K., & McIntosh, A.R. (2002). Aging gracefully: Compensatory brain activity in high-performing older adults. *NeuroImage, 17*(3), 1394-1402.

Cabeza, R., Anderson, N.D., Locantore, J.K., & McIntosh, A.R. (2002). Aging gracefully: Compensatory brain activity in high-performing older adults. *NeuroImage, 17*(3), 1394-1402.

Cahn-Weiner, D.A., Boyle, P.A., & Malloy, P.F. (2002). Tests of executive function predict instrumental activities of daily living in community-dwelling older individuals. *Applied Neuropsychology, 9*(3), 187-191.

Caligiuri, M.P., & Ellwanger, J. (2000). Motor and cognitive aspects of motor retardation in depression. *Journal of Affective Disorders, 57*(1-3), 83-93.

Caligiuri, M.P., Peavy, G., & Galasko, D.R. (2001). Extrapyramidal signs and cognitive abilities in Alzheimer's disease. *International Journal of Geriatric Psychiatry, 16*(9), 907-911.

Callen, D.J.A., Black, S.E., Gao, F., & Caldwell, C.B. (2002). Limbic system perfusion in Alzheimer's disease measured by MRI-coregistered HMPAO SPET. *European Journal of Nuclear Medicine and Molecular Imaging, 29*(7), 899-906.

Camarda, R., Camarda, C., Monastero, R., Grimaldi, S., Camarda, L.K., Pipia, C., ... Gangitano, M. (2007). Movements execution in amnestic mild cognitive impairment and Alzheimer's Disease. *Behavioural Neurology, 18*(3), 135-142.

Cape, E.G., & Jones, B.E. (1998). Differential modulation of high-frequency electroencephalogram activity and sleep-wake state by noradrenaline and serotonin microinjections into the region of cholinergic basalis neurons. *Journal of Neuroscience, 18*(7), 2653-2666.

Casey, B.J., Castellanos, F.X., Giedd, J.H., Marsh, W.L., Hamburger, S.D., Schubert, A.B., & Rapoport, J.L. (1997). Implication of right frontostriatal circuitry in response inhibition and attention-deficit/hyperactivity disorder. *Journal of the American Academy of Child & Adolescent Psychiatry, 36*(3), 374-383.

Casey, B.J., Thomas, K.M., Davidson, M.C., Kunz, K., & Franzen, P.L. (2002). Dissociating striatal and hippocampal function developmentally with a stimulus-response compatibility task. *Journal of Neuroscience, 22*(19), 8647–8652.

Casey, K.L., Lorenz, J., & Minoshima, S. (2003). Insights into the pathophysiology of neuropathic pain through functional brain imaging. *Experimental Neurology, 184*(Suppl. 1), S80-S88.

Castellani, R.J., Smith, M.A., Perry, G., & Friedland, R.P. (2004). Cerebral amyloid angiopathy: Major contributor or decorative response to Alzheimer's disease pathogenesis. *Neurobiology of Aging, 25*(5), 599-602.

Catani, M., Howard, R.J., Pajevic, S., & Jones, D.K. (2002). Virtual in vivo interactive dissection of white matter fasciculi in the human brain. *NeuroImage, 17*(1), 77–94.

Cerf-Ducastel, B., & Murphy, C. (2003). FMRI brain activation in response to odors is reduced in primary olfactory areas of elderly subjects. *Brain Research, 986*(1-2), 39-53.

Chan, D., Fox, N.C., Scahill, R.I., Crum, W.R., Whitwell, J.L., Leschziner, G., & Rossor, M.N. (2001). Patterns of temporal lobe atrophy in semantic dementia and Alzheimer's disease. *Annals of Neurology, 49*(4), 433-442.

Chen, L.C., Metcalfe, J.S., Chang, T.Y., Jeka, J.J., & Clark, J.E. (2008). The development of infant upright posture: sway less or sway differently? *Experimental Brain Research, 186*(2), 293-303.

Chen, P., Ratcliff, G., Belle, S.H., Cauley, J.A., DeKosky, S.T., & Ganguli, M. (2000). Cognitive tests that best discriminate between presymptomatic AD and those who remain nondemented. *Neurology, 55*(12), 1847-1853.

Cheron, G., Bouillot, E., Dan, B., Bengoetxea, A., Draye, J.P., & Lacquaniti, F. (2001). Development of a kinematic coordination pattern in toddler locomotion: Planar covariation. *Experimental Brain Research, 137*(3 4), 455 466.

Chetelat, G., & Baron, J.C. (2003). Early diagnosis of Alzheimer's disease: Contribution of structural neuroimaging. *NeuroImage, 18*(2), 525-541.

Chibnall, J.T., & Tait, R.C. (2001). Pain assessment in cognitively impaired and unimpaired older adults: a comparison of four scales. *Pain, 92*(1-2), 173-186.

Chinta, S.J., & Andersen, J.K. (2005). Dopaminergic neurons. *The International Journal of Biochemistry & Cell Biology, 37*(5), 942-946.

Chong, R.K., Horak, F.B., Frank, J., & Kaye, J. (1999). Sensory organization for balance: specific deficits in Alzheimer's but not in Parkinson's disease. *Journals of Gerontology Series A-Biological Sciences and Medical Sciences, 54*(3), M122-M128.

Choudburry, S., Charman, T., Bird, V., & Blakemore, S.J. (2007). Development of action representation during adolescence. *Neuropsychologia, 45*(2), 255-262.

Christensen, H., Mackinnon, A.J., Korten, A., & Jorm, A.F. (2001). The 'common cause hypothesis' of cognitive aging: Evidence for not only a common factor but also specific associations of age with vision and grip strength in a cross-sectional analysis. *Psychology and Aging, 16*(4), 588-599.

Christensen, M.S., Lundbye-Jensen, J., Geertsen, S.S., Petersen, T.H., Paulson, O.B., & Nielsen, J.B. (2007). Premotor cortex modulates somatosensory cortex during voluntary movements without proprioceptive feedback. *Nature Neuroscience, 10*(4), 417-419.

Chudler, E.H., & Dong, W.K. (1995). The role of the basal ganglia in nociception and pain. *Pain, 60* (1), 3-38.

Churchill, J.D., Galvez, R., Colcombe, S., Swain, R.A., Kramer, A.F., & Greenough, W.T. (2002). Exercise, experience and the aging brain. *Neurobiology of Aging, 23*(5), 941-955.

Churchill, J.D., Stanis, J.J., Press, C., Kushelev, M., & Greenough, W.T. (2003). Is procedural memory relatively spared from age effects? *Neurobiology of Aging, 24*(6), 883-892.

Ciccarelli, O., Toosy, A.T., Marsden, J.F., Wheeler-Kingshott, C.M., Sahyoun, C., Matthews, P.M., ... Thompson, A.J. (2005). Identifying brain regions for integrative sensorimotor processing with ankle movements. *Experimental Brain Research, 166*(1), 31-42.

Clare, L., & Woods, B. (2003). Cognitive rehabilitation and cognitive training for early-stage Alzheimer's disease and vascular dementia. *Cochrane Database of Systematic Reviews, 4*, CD003260.

Claxton, L.J., Keen, R., & McCarty, M.E. (2003). Evidence of motor planning in infant reaching behavior. *Psychological Science, 14*(4), 354-356.

Closs, S.J., Barr, B., Briggs, M., Cash, K., & Seers, K. (2004). A comparison of five pain assessment scales for nursing home residents with varying degrees of cognitive impairment. *Journal of Pain and Symptom Management, 27*(3), 196-205.

Coffey, C.E., Wilkinson, W.E., Parashos, I.A., Soady, S.A.R., Sullivan, R.J. Patterson, L.J., & Djang, W.T. (1992). Quantitative cerebral anatomy of the aging human brain: A cross sectional study using magnetic resonance imaging. *Neurology, 42*(30), 527-536.

Cohen, G.D., & Havlik, R.J. (1993). Epidemiology of aging comes of age. *Annals of Epidemiology 3*(4), 448-450.

Cohen-Mansfield, J., & Werner, P. (1999). Longitudinal predictors of non-aggressive agitated behaviors in the elderly. *International Journal of Geriatric Psychiatry, 14*(10), 831-844.

Cohn, E.S. (1999). Hearing loss with aging. *Clinics in Geriatric Medicine, 15*(1), 145-161.

Colcombe, S., & Kramer, A.F. (2003). Fitness effects on the cognitive function of older adults: A meta-analytic study. *Psychological Science 14*(2), 125-130.

Colcombe, S.J., Erickson, K.I., Raz, N., Webb, A.G., Cohen, N.J., McAuley, E., & Kramer, A.F. (2003). Aerobic fitness reduces brain tissue loss in aging humans. *Journals of Gerontology Series A-Biological Sciences and Medical Sciences, 58*(2), 176-180.

Colcombe, S.J., Kramer, A.F., Erickson, K.I., Scalf, P., McAuley, E., Cohen, N.J., ... Elavsky, S. (2004). Cardiovascular fitness, cortical plasticity, and aging. *Proceedings of the National Academy of Sciences of the United States of America, 101*(9), 3316-3321.

Coleman, P.D., & Flood, D.G. (1987). Neuron numbers and dendritic extent in normal aging and Alzheimer's disease. *Neurobiology of Aging, 8*(6), 521-545.

Collie, A., & Maruff, P. (2000). The neuropsychology of preclinical Alzheimer's disease and mild cognitive impairment. *Neuroscience and Biobehavioral Reviews, 24*(3), 365-374.

Corbin, S.L., & Eastwood, M.R. (1986). Sensory deficits and mental disorders of old age: Causal or coincidental associations? *Psychological Medicine, 16*(2),251-256.

Cott, C.A., Dawson, P., Sidani, T., & Wells, T. (2002). The effects of a walking/talking program on communication, ambulation, and functional status in residents with Alzheimer disease. *Alzheimer Disease & Associated Disorders, 16*(2), 81-87.

Cotter, V.T. (2005). Restraint free care in older adults with dementia. *Keio Journal of Medicine, 54*(2), 80-84.

Court, J.A., & Perry, E.K. (2003). Neurotransmitter abnormalities in vascular dementia. *International Psychogeriatrics,15*(Suppl. 1), 81-87.

Cousins, D.A., Burton, E.J., Burn, D., Gholkar, A., McKeith, I.G., & O'Brien, J.T. (2003). Atrophy of the putamen in dementia with Lewy bodies but not Alzheimer's disease: An MRI study. *Neurology, 61*(9), 1191-1195.

Cummings, J.L., & Back, C. (1998). The cholinergic hypothesis of neuropsychiatric symptoms in Alzheimer's disease. *The American Journal of Geriatric Psychiatry, 6*(2), S64-S78.

Cummings, J.L., & Benson, D.F. (1984). Subcortical dementia. Review of an emerging concept. *Archives of Neurology, 41*(8), 874-879.

Cunnington, R., Windischberger, C., & Moser, E. (2005). Premovement activity of the pre-supplementary motor area and the readiness for action: Studies of time-resolved event-related functional MRI. *Human Movement Science, 24*(5-6), 644-656.

D'Angelo, E., & de Zeeuw, C.I. (2009). Timing and plasticity in the cerebellum: Focus on the granular layer. *Trends in Neuroscience, 32*(1), 30-40.

Dagres, N., Saller, B., Haude, M., Hüsing, J., von Birgelen, C., Schmermund, A., ... Erbel, R. (2004). Insulin sensitivity and coronary vasoreactivity: insulin sensitivity relates to adenosine-stimulated coronary flow response in human subjects. *Clinical Endocrinology, 61*(6), 724-731.

Dastoor, D., Schwartz, G., & Kurzman, D. (1991). Clock-drawing: An assessment technique in dementia. *Journal of Clinical and Experimental Gerontology, 13*(1-2), 69-85.

Davies, R.R., Graham, K.S., Xuereb, J.H., Williams, G.B., & Hodges, J.R. (2004). The human perirhinal cortex and semantic memory. *European Journal of Neuroscience, 20*(9), 2441-2446.

Davies, R.R., Hodges, J.R., Krill, J.J., Patterson, K., Halliday, G.M., & Xuereb, J.H. (2005). The pathological basis of semantic dementia. *Brain 128*, 1984-1995.

de Bruin, E.D., Swanenburg, J., Betschon, E., & Murer, K. (2009). A randomised controlled trial investigating motor skill training as a function of attentional focus in old age. *BMC Geriatrics, 9* (15), 15.

de Groot, J.C., de Leeuw, F.-E., Oudkerk, M., Hofman, A., Jolles, J., & Breteler, M.M.B. (2001). Cerebral white matter lesions and subjective cognitive dysfunction. The Rotterdam Scan Study. *Neurology, 56*(11), 1539-1545.

de Groot, J.C., de Leeuw, F.-E., Oudkerk, M., van Gijn, J., Hofman, A., Jolles, J., & Breteler, M.M.B. (2002). Periventricular cerebral white matter lesions predict rate of cognitive decline. *Annals of Neurology, 52*(3), 335-341.

de Knegt, N., & Scherder, E.J.A. (2011). Pain in adults with intellectual disabilities. *Pain, 152*(5), 971-974.

de Leeuw, F.-E., de Groot, J.C., Oudkerk, M., Witteman, J.C.M., Hofman, A., van Gijn, J., & Breteler, M.M.B. (2002). Hypertension and cerebral white matter lesions in a prospective cohort study. *Brain, 125*, 765-772.

de Mendonça, A., Ribeiro, F., Guerreiro, M., & Garcia, C. (2004). Frontotemporal mild cognitive impairment. *Journal of Alzheimer's Disease, 6*(1), 1-9.

Debaere, F., Swinnen, S.P., Béatse, E., Sunaert, S., Van Hecke, P., & Duysens J. (2001). Brain areas involved in interlimb coordination: a distributed network. *Neuroimage, 14*(5), 947-58

DeCarli, C., Murphy, D.G.M., Gillette, J.A., Haxby, J.V., Teichberg, D., Schapiro, M.B., & Horwitz, B. (1994). Lack of age-related differences in temporal lobe volume of very healthy adults. *American Journal of Neuroradiology, 15*(4), 689-696.

Della Sala, S., Francescani, A., & Spinnler, H. (2002). Gait apraxia after bilateral supplementary motor area lesion. *Journal of Neurology, Neurosurgery and Psychiatry, 72*(1), 77-85.

den Heijer, T., Launer, L.J., Prins, N.D., van Dijk, E.J., Vermeer, S.E., Hofman, A., & Breteler, M.M. (2005). Association between blood pressure, white matter lesions, and atrophy of the medial temporal lobe. *Neurology, 64*(2), 263-267.

Desmond, D.W. (2004). The neuropsychology of vascular cognitive impairment: Is there a specific cognitive deficit? *Journal of the Neurological Sciences, 226*(1-2), 3-7.

Desrosiers, J., Hébert, R., Bravo, G., & Rochette, A. (1999). Age-related changes in upper extremity performance of elderly people: A longitudinal study. *Experimental Gerontology, 34*(3), 393-405.

Diamond, A. (2000). Close interrelation of motor development and cognitive development and of the cerebellum and prefrontal cortex. *Child Development, 71*(1), 44-56.

Diaz, M., Sailor, K., Cheung, D., & Kuslansky, G. (2004). Category size effects in semantic and letter fluency in Alzheimer's patients. *Brain and Language, 89*(1), 108-114.

Dick, M.B., Hsieh, S., Dick-Muehlke, C., Davis, D.S., & Cotman, C.W. (2000). The variability of practice hypothesis in motor learning: Does it apply to Alzheimer's disease? *Brain and Cognition, 44*(3), 470-489.

Dickin, D.C., & Rose, D.J. (2004). Sensory organization abilities during upright stance in late-onset Alzheimer's-type dementia. *Experimental Aging Research, 30*(4), 373-390.

Diehl-Schmid, J., Grimmer, T., Drzezga, A., Bornschein, S., Riemenschneider, M., Förstl, H., ... Kurz, A. (2007). Decline of cerebral glucose metabolism in frontotemporal dementia: A longitudinal 18F-FDG-PET-study. *Neurobiology of Aging, 28*(1), 42-50.

Diener, H.C., & Dichgans, J. (1992). Pathophysiology of cerebellar ataxia. *Movement Disorders, 7*(2), 95-109.

Dirnberger, G., Frith, C.D., & Jahanshahi, M. (2005). Executive dysfunction in Parkinson's disease is associated with altered pallidal-frontal processing. *NeuroImage, 25*(2), 588-599.

Drachman, D.A. (1997). Aging and the brain: A new frontier. *Annals of Neurology, 42*(6), 819-828.

Driscoll, I., Hamilton, D.A., Petropoulos, H., Yeo, R.A., Brooks, W.M., Baumgartner, R.N., & Sutherland, R.J. (2003). The aging hippocampus: Cognitive, biochemical and structural findings. *Cerebral Cortex, 13*(12), 1344-1351.

Du, A., Schuff, N., Chao, L.L., Kornak, J., Ezekiel, F., Jagust, W.J., & Weiner, M.W. (2005). White matter lesions are associated with cortical atrophy more than entorhinal and hippocampal atrophy. *Neurobiology of Aging, 26*(4), 553-559.

Du, A.T., Schuff, N., Kramer, J.H., Rosen, H.J., Gorno-Tempini, M.L., Rankin, K., ... Weiner, M.W. (2007). Different regional patterns of cortical thinning in Alzheimer's disease and frontotemporal dementia. *Brain, 130*, 1159-1166.

Dubois, J., Hertz-Pannier, L., Dehaene-Lambertz, G., Cointepas, Y., & Le Bihan, D. (2006). Assessment of the early organization and maturation of infants' cerebral white matter fiber bundles: a feasibility study using quantitative diffusion tensor imaging and tractography. *Neuroimage 30(4)*, 1121-1132.

Duke, L.M., & Kaszniak, A.W. (2000). Executive control functions in degenerative dementias: A comparative review. *Neuropsychology Review, 10*(2), 75-99.

Dunnett, S.B., & Fibiger, H.C. (1993). Role of forebrain cholinergic systems in learning and memory: Relevance to the cognitive deficits of aging and Alzheimer's dementia. *Progress in Brain Research, 98*, 413-420.

Dunsky, A., Dickstein, R., Ariav, C., Deutsch, J., & Marcovitz, E. (2006). Motor imagery practice in gait rehabilitation of chronic post-stroke hemiparesis: Four case studies. *International Journal of Rehabilitation Research, 29*(4), 351-356.

Ebeling, U., & von Cramon, D. (1992). Topography of the uncinate fascicle and adjacent temporal fiber tracts. *Acta Neurochirurgia, 115*(3-4), 143-148.

Economou, A., Papageorgiou, S.G., Karageorgiou, C., & Vassilopoulos, D. (2007). Nonepisodic memory deficits in amnestic MCI. *Cognitive & Behavioral Neurology, 20*(2), 99-106.

Edwards-Lee, T., Miller, B.L., Benson, D.F., Cumings, J.L., Russell, G.L., Boone, K., & Mena, I. (1997). The temporal variant of frontotemporal dementia. *Brain, 120,* 1027-1040.

Eggermont, L.H., Swaab, D.F., Hol, E.M., & Scherder, E.J. (2009). Walking the line: a randomised trial on the effects of a short term walking programme on cognition in dementia *Journal of Neurology, Neurosurgery and Psychiatry, 80*(7), 802-804.

Eggermont, L.H.P., Swaab, D.F., Luiten., P.G.M., & Scherder, E.J.A. (2006). Exercise, cognition and Alzheimer's disease: More is not necessarily better. *Neuroscience and Behavioral Reviews, 30*(4), 562-575.

Ehrsson, H.H., Fagergren, E., & Forssberg, H. (2001). Differential fronto-parietal activation depending on force used in a precision grip task: An fMRI study. *Journal of Neurophysiology, 85*(6), 2613-2623.

Ekman, P., & Friesen, W. (1978). *Investigator's guide to Facial Action Coding System.* Palo Alto, Consulting Psychologists Press.

Eldridge, L.L., Engel, S.A., Zeineh, M.M., Bookheimer, S.Y., & Knowlton, B.J. (2005). A dissociation of encoding and retrieval processes in the human hippocampus. *Journal of Neuroscience, 25*(13), 3280-3286.

Elsinger, C.L., Rao, S.M., Zimbelman, J.L., Reynolds, N.C., Blindauer, K.A., & Hoffmann, R.G. (2003). Neural basis for impaired time reproduction in Parkinson's disease: An fMRI study. *Journal of the International Neuropsychological Society, 9*(7), 1088-98.

Eluvathingal, T.J., Hasan, K.M., Kramer, L., Fletcher, J.M., & Ewing-Cobbs, L. (2007). Quantitative diffusion tensor tractography of association and projection fibers in normally developing children and adolescents. *Cerebral Cortex, 17*(12), 2760-2768.

Emre, M. (2003). Dementia associated with Parkinson's disease. *Lancet Neurology, 2*(4), 229-237.

Engelborghs, S., & DeDeyn, P.P. (1997). The neurochemistry of Alzheimer's disease. *Acta Neurologica, 97*(2), 67-84.

Enoch, J.M., Werner, J.S., Haegerstrom-Portnoy, G., Lakshminarayanan, V., & Rynders, M. (1999). Forever young: Visual functions not affected or minimally affected by aging. A review. *Journal of Gerontology: Biological Sciences, 54*(8), B336-B351.

Enrietto, J.A., Jacobsen, K.M., & Baloh, R.W. (1999). Aging effects on auditory and vestibular responses: A longitudinal study. *American Journal of Otolaryngology. 20*(6), 371-8.

Erickson, C.A., & Barnes, C.A. (2003). The neurobiology of memory changes in normal aging. *Experimental Gerontology, 38*(1-2), 61-69.

Eshel, N., Nelson, E.E., Blair, R.J., Pine, D.S., & Ernst, M. (2007). Neural substrates of choice selection in adults and adolescents: Development of the ventrolateral prefrontal and anterior cingulate cortices. *Neuropsychologia, 45*(6), 1270-1279.

Esiri, M.M., Pearson, R.C.A., & Powell, T.P.S. (1986). The cortex of the primary auditory area in Alzheimer's disease. *Brain Research, 366*(1-2), 385-387.

Eslinger, P.J., Moore, P., Troiani, V., Antani, S., Cross, K., Kwok, S., & Grossman, M. (2007). Oops! Resolving social dilemmas in frontotemporal dementia. *Journal of Neurology, Neurosurgery & Psychiatry, 78*(5), 157-160.

Esposito, G., Kirkby, B.S., Van Horn, J.D., Ellmore, T.M., & Berman, K.F. (1999). Context-dependent, neural system-specific neurophysiological concomitants of ageing: Mapping PET correlates during cognitive activation. *Brain, 122,* 963-979.

Evans, D.A., Funkenstein, H., Alberts, M.S., Scherr, P.A., Cook, N.R., Chown, M.J., & Taylor, J.O. (1989). Prevalence of Alzheimer's disease in a community population of older persons. Higher than previously reported. *Journal of the American Medical Association, 262*(18), 2551-2556.

Evans, E.M., Racette, S.B., Peterson, L.R., Villareal, D.T., Greiwe, J.S., & Holloszy, J.O. (2005). Aerobic power and insulin action improve in response to endurance exercise training in healthy 77-87 yr olds. *Journal of Applied Physiology, 98*(1), 40-45.

Ezrin-Waters, C., & Resch, L. (1986). The nucleus basalis of Meynert. *Canadian Journal of Neurological Sciences, 13*(1), 8-14.

Fabbro, F., Clarici, A., & Bava, A. (1996). Effects of left basal ganglia lesions on language production. *Perceptual and Motor Skills, 82*(3), 1291-1298.

Fabre, C., Chamari, K., Mucci, P., Masse-Biron, J., & Prefaut, C. (2002). Improvement of cognitive function by mental and/or individualized aerobic training in healthy elderly subjects. *International Journal of Sports Medicine, 23*(6), 415-421.

Farrell, M.J., Katz, B., & Helme, R.D. (1996). The impact of dementia on the pain experience. *Pain, 67* (1), 7-15.

Fassbender, C., Murphy, K., Foxe, J.J., Wylie, G.R., Javitt, D.C., Robertson, I.H., & Garavan, H. (2004). A topography of executive functions and their interactions revealed by functional magnetic resonance imaging. *Cognitive Brain Research, 20*(2), 132-143.

Feldt, K. (2001). The checklist of nonverbal pain indicators (CNPI). *Pain Management Nursing, 1*(1), 13-21.

Fernando, M.S., & Ince, P.G. (2004). Vascular pathologies and cognition in a population-based cohort of elderly people. *Journal of the Neurological Sciences, 226*(1-2), 13-17.

Ferrell, B.A., Ferrell, B.R., & Rivera, L. (1995). Pain in cognitively impaired nursing home patients. *Journal of Pain and Symptom Management, 10*(8), 591-598.

Filley, C.M. (1998). The behavioral neurology of cerebral white matter. *Neurology, 50*(6), 1535-1540.

Fisher-Morris, M., & Gellatly, A. (1997). The experience and expression of pain in Alzheimer patients. *Age and Ageing, 26*(6), 497-500.

Florin-Lechner, S.M., Druhan, J.P., Aston-Jones, G., & Valentino, R.J. (1996). Enhanced norepinephrine release in prefrontal cortex with burst stimulation of the local coeruleus. *Brain Research, 742*(1-2), 89-97.

Floyer-Lea, A., & Matthews, P.M. (2004). Changing brain networks for visuomotor control with increased movement automaticity. *Journal of Neurophysiology,. 92*(4), 2405-2412.

Folstein, M., Folstein, S., & McHugh, P. (1975). 'Mini-Mental State': A practical method for grading the cognitive state of patients for the clinician. *Journal of Psychiatric Research, 12*(3), 189-198.

Ford, B. (1998). Pain in Parkinson's disease. *Clinical Neuroscience, 5*(2), 63-72.

Fossati, P., Radtchenko, A., & Boyer, P. (2004). Neuroplasticity: From MRI to depressive symptoms. *European Neuropsychopharmacology, 14*, S503-S510.

Foundas, A.L., Leonard, C.M., Mahoney, S.M., Agee, O.F., & Heilman, K.M. (1997). Atrophy of the hippocampus, parietal cortex, and insula in Alzheimer's disease: A volumetric magnetic resonance imaging study. *Neuropsychiatry, Neuropsychology and Behavioral Neurology, 10*(2), 81-89.

Fox, N.C., Warrington, E.K., Freeborough, P.A., Hartikainen, P., Kennedy, A.M., Stevens, J.M., & Rossor, M.N. (1996). Presymptomatic hippocampal atrophy in Alzheimer's disease. A longitudinal MRI study. *Brain, 119*, 2001-2007.

Francese, T., Sorrell, J., & Butler, F.R. (1997). The effects of regular exercise on muscle strength and functional abilities of late stage Alzheimer's residents. *American Journal of Alzheimer's Disease, 12*, 122-127.

Franchesi, M., Anchisi, D., Pelati, O., Zuffi, M., Matarrese, M., Moresco, R.M., & Perani, D. (2005). Glucose metabolism and serotonin receptors in the frontotemporal lobe degeneration. *Annals of Neurology, 57*(2), 216-225.

Franssen, E.H., Souren, L.E., Torossian, C.L., & Reisberg, B. (1999). Equilibrium and limb coordination in mild cognitive impairment and mild Alzheimer's disease. *Journal of the American Geriatrics Society, 47*(4), 463-469.

Fratiglioni, L., Paillard-Borg, S., & Winblad, B. (2004). An active and socially integrated lifestyle in late life might protect against dementia. *Lancet Neurology, 3*(6), 343-353.

Frederiksen, H., Hjelmborg, J., Mortensen, J., McGue, M., Vaupel, J.W., & Christensen, K. (2006). Age trajectories of grip strength: Cross-sectional and longitudinal data among 8,342 Danes aged 46-102. *Annals of Epidemiology, 16*(7), 554-562.

Freedman, M., & Oscar-Berman, M. (1987). Tactile discrimination learning deficits in Alzheimer's and Parkinson's diseases. *Archives of Neurology, 44*(4), 394-398.

Friedman, R., & Tappen, R.M. (1991). The effect of planned walking on communication in Alzheimer's disease. *Journal of the American Geriatrics Society, 39*(7), 650-654.

Frisina, D.R., & Frisina, R.D. (1997). Speech recognition in noise and presbycusis: Relations to possible neural mechanisms. *Hearing Research, 106*(1-2), 95-104.

Frisoni, G.B., Galluzzi, S., Bresciani, L., Zanetti, O., & Geroldi, C. (2002). Mild cognitive impairment with subcortical vascular features: Clinical characteristics and outcome. *Journal of Neurology, 249* (10), 1423-1432.

Frisoni, G.B., Pievani, M., Testa, C., Sabattoli, F., Bresciani, L., Bonetti, M., ... Thompson, P.M. (2007). The topography of grey matter involvement in early and late onset Alzheimer's disease. *Brain, 130*, 720-730.

Frisoni, G.B., Prestia, A., Rasser, P.E., Bonetti, M., & Thompson, P.M. (2009). In vivo mapping of incremental cortical atrophy from incipient to overt Alzheimer's disease. *Journal of Neurology, 256*(6), 916-924.

Fuchs-Lacelle, S., & Hadjistavropoulos, T. (2004). Development and preliminary validation of the pain assessment checklist for seniors with limited ability to communicate (PACSLAC). *Pain Management Nursing, 5*(1), 37-49.

Fukunaga, A., Uematsu, H., & Sugimoto, K. (2005). Influences of aging on taste perception and oral somatic sensation. *Journal of Gerontology: Medical Sciences, 60A*(1), 109-113.

Fukuyama, H., Ouchi, Y., Matsuzaki, S., Nagahama, Y., Yamauchi, H., Ogawa, M., ... Shibasaki, H. (1997). Brain functional activity during gait in normal subjects: A SPECT study. *Neuroscience Letters, 228*(3), 183-186.

Funkenstein, H.H., Albert, M.S., Cook, N.R., West, C.G., Scherr, P.A., Chown, M.J., & Evans, D.A. (1993). Extrapyramidal signs and other neurologic findings in clinically diagnosed Alzheimer's disease. *Archives of Neurology, 50*(1), 51-56.

Fuster, J.M. (2002). Frontal lobe and cognitive development. *Journal of Neurocytology, 31*(3-5), 373-385.

Garcia-Alloza, M., Gill-Bea, F.J., Diez-Ariza, M., Chen, C.P.L.-H., Francis, P.T., Lasheras, B., & Ramirez, M.J. (2005). Cholinergic-serotonergic imbalance contributes to cognitive and behavioural symptoms in Alzheimer's disease. *Neuropsychologia, 43*(3), 442-449.

García-Cabezas, M.A., Rico, B., Sánchez-González, M.A., & Cavada, C. (2007). Distribution of the dopamine innervation in the macaque and human thalamus. *NeuroImage, 34*(3), 965-984.

Garraux, G., Salmon, E., Degueldre, C., Lemaire, C., Laureys, S., & Franck, G. (1999). Comparison of impaired subcortico-frontal metabolic networks in normal aging, subcortico-frontal dementia, and cortical frontal dementia. *NeuroImage, 10*(2), 149-162.

Gasser, T., Rousson, V., Caflisch, J., & Largo, R. (2007). Quantitative reference curves for associated movements in children and adolescents. *Developmental Medicine & Child Neurology, 49*(8), 608-614.

Geddes, J.W., & Cotman, C.W. (1991). Plasticity in Alzheimer's disease: Too much or not enough? *Neurobiology of Aging, 12*(4), 330-333.

Gerber, D.J., Sotnikova, T.D., Gainetdinov, R.R., Huang, S.Y., Caron, M.G., & Tonegawa, S. (2001). Hyperactivity, elevated dopaminergic transmission, and response to amphetamine in M1 muscarinic acetylcholine receptor-deficient mice. *Proceedings of the National Academy of Sciences of the United States of America, 98*(26), 15312-15317.

Ghilardi, M.F., Alberoni, M., Marelli, S., Rossi, M., Franceschi, M., Ghez, C., & Fazio, F. (1999). Impaired movement control in Alzheimer's disease. *Neuroscience Letters, 260*(1), 45-48.

Gibson, S.J., Voukelatos, X., Ames, D., Flicker, L., & Helme, R.D. (2001). An examination of pain perception and cerebral event-related potentials following carbon dioxide laser stimulation in patients with Alzheimer's disease and age-matched control volunteers. *Pain Research & Management, 6*(3), 126-132.

Gilboa, A., Ramirez, J., Köhler, S., Westmacott, R., Black, S.E., & Moscovitch, M. (2005). Retrieval of autobiographical memory in Alzheimer's disease: Relation to volumes of medial temporal lobe and other structures. *Hippocampus, 15*(4), 535-550.

Gill, T.M., & Gallagher, M. (1998). Evaluation of muscarinic M2 receptor sites in basal forebrain and brainstem cholinergic systems of behaviorally characterized young and aged Long-Evans rats. *Neurobiology of Aging, 19*(3), 217-225.

Gilles, M.A., & Wing, A.M. (2003). Age-related changes in grip force and dynamics of hand movement. *Journal of Motor Behavior, 35*(1), 79-85.

Gilmore, G.C., Wenk, H.E., Naylor, L.A., & Koss, E. (1994). Motion perception and Alzheimer's disease. *Journal of Gerontology, 49*(2), 52-57.

Giorgio, A., Watkins, K.E., Douaud, G., James, A.C., James, S., De Stefano, N., ... Johansen-Berg, H. (2008). Changes in white matter microstructure during adolescence. *NeuroImage, 39*(1), 52-61.

Gogtay, N., Giedd, J.N., Lusk, L., Hayashi, K.M., Greenstein, D., Vaituzis, A.C., ... Thompson, P.M. (2004). Dynamic mapping of human cortical development during childhood through early adulthood. *Proceedings of the National Academy of Sciences of the United States of America, 101*(21), 8174-8179.

Gold, B.T., Balota, D.A., Kirchhoff, B.A., & Buckner, R.L. (2005). Common and dissociable activation patterns associated with controlled semantic and phonological processing: Evidence from fMRI adaptation. *Cerebral Cortex, 15*(9), 1438-1450.

Goldman, W.P., Baty, J.D., Buckles, V.D., Sahrmann, S., & Morris, J.C. (1999). Motor dysfunction in mildly demented AD individuals without extrapyramidal signs. *Neurology, 53*(5), 956-962.

Gotz, J., Schild, A., Hoerndli, F., & Pennanen, L. (2004). Amyloid-induced neurofibrillary tangle formation in Alzheimer's disease: Insight from transgenic mouse and tissue-culture models. *International Journal of Developmental Neuroscience, 22*(7), 453-465.

Grady, C.L., Furey, M.L., Pietrini, P., Horwitz, B., & Rapoport, S.I. (2001). Altered brain functional connectivity and impaired short-term memory in Alzheimer's disease. *Brain, 124,* 739-756.

Grady, C.L., McIntosh, A.R., & Craik, F.I.M. (2003). Age-related differences in the functional connectivity of the hippocampus during memory encoding. *Hippocampus, 13*(5), 572-586.

Grady, C.L., McIntosh, A.R., Beig, S., Keightley, M.L., Burian, H., & Black, S.E. (2003). Evidence from functional neuroimaging of a compensatory prefrontal network in Alzheimer's disease. *The Journal of Neuroscience, 23*(3), 986-993.

Graham, N.L., Emery, T., & Hodges, J.R. (2004). Distinctive cognitive profiles in Alzheimer's disease and subcortical vascular dementia. *Journal of Neurology, Neurosurgery and Psychiatry, 75*(1), 61-71.

Grau-Olivares, M., Bartrés-Faz, D., Arboix, A., Soliva, J.C., Rovira, M., Targa, C., & Junqué, C. (2007). Mild cognitive impairment after lacunar infarction: Voxel-based morphometry and neuropsychological assessment. *Cerebrovasculair Diseases, 23*(5-6), 353-361.

Greenamyre, J.T. (1991). Neuronal bioenergetic defects, excitotoxicity and Alzheimer's disease: 'Use it or lose it'. *Neurobiology of Aging, 12*(4), 334-336.

Grieve, S.M., Williams, L.M., Paul, R.H., Clark, C.R., & Gordon, E. (2007). Cognitive aging, executive function, and fractional anisotropy: A diffusion tensor MR imaging study. *American Journal of Neuroradiology, 28*(2), 226-235.

Grön, G., & Riepe, M.W. (2004). Neural basis for the cognitive continuum in episodic memory from health to Alzheimer disease. *American Journal of Geriatric Psychiatry, 12*(8), 648-652.

Grön, G., Brandenburg, I., Wunderlich, A.P., & Riepe, M.W. (2006). Inhibition of hippocampal function in mild cognitive impairment: Targeting the cholinergic hypothesis. *Neurobiology of Aging, 27*(1), 78-87.

Grossi, D., Fragassi, N.A., Chiacchio, L., Valoroso, L., Tuccillo, R., Perrotta, C., ... Trojano, L., (2002). Do visuospatial and constructional disturbances differentiate frontal variant of frontotemporal dementia and Alzheimer's disease? An experimental study of a clinical belief. *International Journal of Geriatric Psychiatry, 17*(4), 641-648.

Grundman, M., Petersen, R.C., Ferris, S.H., Thomas, R.G., Aisen, P.S., Bennett, D.A., Thal, L.J. (2004). Mild cognitive impairment can be distinguished from Alzheimer disease and normal aging for clinical trials. *Archives of Neurology, 61*(1), 59-66.

Guarch, J., Marcos, T., Salamero, M., & Blesa, R. (2004). Neuropsychological markers of dementia in patients with memory complaints. *International Journal of Geriatric Psychiatry, 19*(4), 352-358.

Guillozet, A.L., Weintraub, S., Mash, D.C., & Mesulam, M. (2003). Neurofibrillary tangles, amyloid, and memory in aging and mild cognitive impairment. *Archives of Neurology, 60*(5), 729-736.

Gunning-Dixon, F.M., & Raz, N. (2000). The cognitive correlates of white matter abnormalities in normal aging: A quantitative review. *Neuropsychology, 14*(2), 224-32.

Gutchess, A.H., Welsh, R.C., Hedden, T., Bangert, A., Minear, M., Liu, L.L., & Park, D.C. (2005). Aging and the neural correlates of successful picture encoding: fontal activations compensate for decreased medial-temporal activity. *Journal of Cognitive Neuroscience, 17*(1), 84-96.

Haas, D.C., Kent, P.F., & Friedman, D.I. (1993). Headache caused by a single lesion of multiple sclerosis in the periaqueductal gray area. *Headache, 33*(8), 452-55.

Hadjistovropoulos, T., LaChapelle, D.L., Hadjistavropoulos, H.D., Green, S., & Asmundson, G.J.G. (2002). Using facial expressions to assess muculoskeletal pain in older persons. *European Journal of Pain, 6*(3), 179-187.

Hageman, P.A., & Thomas, V.S. (2002). Gait performance in dementia: The effects of a 6-week resistance training program in an adult day-care setting. *International Journal of Geriatric Psychiatry, 17*(4), 329-334.

Hall, J.R., & Harvey, M.B. (2008). Behavioral regulation: Factor analysis and application of the Behavioral Dyscontrol Scale in dementia and mild cognitive impairment. *International Journal of Geriatric Psychiatry, 23*(3), 314-318.

Halliday, G.M., Double, K.L., Macdonald, V., & Kril, J.J. (2003). Identifying severely atrophic cortical subregions in Alzheimer's disease. *Neurobiology of Aging, 24*(6), 797-806.

Halper, J., Kennedy, P., Miller, C.M., Morgante, L., Namey, M., & Ross, A.P. (2003). Rethinking cognitive function in multiple sclerosis: A nursing perspective. *The Journal of Neuroscience Nursing, 35*(2), 70-81.

Hanakawa, T., Katsumi, Y., Fukuyama, H., Honda, M., Hayashi, T., Kimura, J., & Shibasaki, H. (1999). Mechanisms underlying gait disturbance in Parkinson's disease: A single photon emission computed tomography study. *Brain, 122*, 1271-1282.

Hanlon, J.T., Landerman, L.R., Wall, W.E., Horner, R.D., Fillenbaum, G.G., Dawson, D.V., ... Blazer, D.G. (1996). Is medication use by community-dwelling elderly people influenced by cognitive function? *Age and Ageing, 25*(3), 190-196.

Harman, D. (1981). The aging process. *Proceedings of the National Academy of Sciences of the United States of America, 78*(11), 7124-7128.

Harwood, D.G., Sultzer, D.L., Feil, D., Monserratt, L., Freedman, E., & Mandelkern, M.A. (2005). Frontal lobe hypometabolism and impaired insight in Alzheimer disease. *American Journal of Geriatric Psychiatry, 13*(11), 934-941.

Hausdorff, J.M., Yogev, G., Springer, S., Simon, E.S., & Giladi, N., (2005). Walking is more like catching than tapping: Gait in the elderly as a complex cognitive task. *Experimental Brain Research, 164* (4), 541-548.

Head, D., Buckner, R.L., Shimony, J.S., Williams, L.E., Akbudak, E., Conturo, T.E., & Snyder, A.Z. (2004). Differential vulnerability of anterior white matter in nondemented aging with minimal acceleration in dementia of the Alzheimer type: Evidence from diffusion tensor imaging. *Cerebral Cortex, 14*(4), 410-423.

Hebert, L.E., Scherr, P.A., McCann, J.J., Bienias, J.L., & Evans, D.A. (2008). Change in direct measures of physical performance among persons with Alzheimer's disease. *Aging & Mental Health, 12*(6), 729-734.

Heft, M.W., Cooper, B.Y., O'Brien, K.K., Hemp, E. & O'Brien, R.. (1996). Aging effects on the perception of noxious and non-noxious thermal stimuli applied to the face. *Aging and Clinical Experimental Research, 8*(1), 35-41.

Heinik, J., Solomesh, I., Raikher, B., & Lin, R. (2002). Can clock drawing test help to differentiate between dementia of the Alzheimer's type and vascular dementia? A preliminary study. *International Journal of Geriatric Psychiatry, 17*(8), 699-703.

Helme, R.D., & Gibson, S.J. (2001). The epidemiology of pain in elderly people. *Clinics in Geriatric Medicine, 17*(3), 417-431.

Herholz, K. (2003). PET studies in dementia. *Annals of Nuclear Medicine, 17*(2), 79-89.

Hermoye, L., Saint-Martin, C., Cosnard, G., Lee, S.K., Kim, J., Nassogne, M.C., … Mori, S. (2006). Pediatric diffusion tensor imaging: Normal database and observation of the white matter maturation in early childhood. *NeuroImage 29*(2), 493-504.

Herr, K., & Decker, S. (2004). Assessment of pain in older adults with severe cognitive impairment. *Annals of Long-Term Care: Clinical Care and Aging, 12*, 46-52.

Herr, K.A., Spratt, K., Mobily, P.R., & Richardson, G. (2004). Pain intensity assessment in older adults. Use of experimental pain to compare psychometric properties and usability of selected pain scales with younger adults. *Clinical Journal of Pain, 20*(4), 207-219.

Herrero, M.T., Barcia, C., & Navarro, J.M. (2002). Functional anatomy of thalamus and basal ganglia. *Child's Nervous System, 18*(8), 386-404.

Heuninckx, S., Wenderoth, N., Debaere, F., Peeters, R., & Swinnen, S.P. (2005). Neural basis of aging: The penetration of cognition into action control. *Journal of Neuroscience, 25*(29), 6787-6796.

Heyder, K., Suchan, B., & Daum, I. (2004). Cortico-subcortical contributions to executive control. *Acta Psychologica, 115*(2-3), 271-289.

Hirao, K., Ohnishi, T., Hirata, Y., Yamashita, F., Mori, T., Moriguchi, Y., … Asada, T. (2005). The prediction of rapid conversion to Alzheimer's disease in mild cognitive impairment using regional blood flow SPECT. *NeuroImage, 28*(4), 1014-1021.

Hirao, K., Ohnishi, T., Matsuda, H., Nemoto, K., Hirata, Y., Yamashita, F., … Iwamoto, T. (2006). Functional interactions between entorhinal cortex and PCC at the very early stage of Alzheimer's disease using brain perfusion single-photon emission computed tomography. *Nuclear Medicine Communications, 27*(2), 151-156.

Hirono, N., Mega, M.S., Dinov, I.D., Mishkin, F., & Cummings, J.L. (2000). Left frontotemporal hypoperfusion is associated with aggression in patients with dementia. *Archives of Neurology, 57*(6), 861-866.

Ho, A.K., Sahakian, B.J., Robbins, T.W., Barker, R.A., Rosser, A.E., & Hodges, J.R. (2002). Verbal fluency in Huntington's disease: A longitudinal analysis of phonemic and semantic clustering and switching. *Neuropsychologia, 40*(8), 1277-1284.

Hodges, J.R. (2001). Frontotemporal dementia (Pick's disease): Clinical features and assessment. *Neurology, 56*(Suppl. 4), S6-S10.

Hof, P.R., & Morrison, J.H. (2004). The aging brain: Morphomolecular senescence of cortical circuits. *Trends in Neurosciences, 27*(10), 607-613.

Höhmann, C., Antuono, P., & Coyle, J.T. (1988). Basal forebrain cholinergic neurons and Alzheimer's disease. In L.L. Iversen, S.D. Iversen & S.H. Snijder (Eds.), *Handbook of Psychofarmacology* (pp. 69-106). New York: Plenum Press.

Horgas, A.L., & Elliott, A.F. (2004). Pain assessment and management in persons with dementia. *Nursing Clinics of North America, 39*(3), 593-606.

Hudson, C.C., & Krebs, D.E. (2000). Frontal plane dynamic stability and coordination in subjects with cerebellar degeneration. *Experimental Brain Research, 132*(1), 103-113.

Huff, F.J., Boller, F., Lucchelli, F., Querriera, R., Beyer, J., & Belle, S. (1987). The neurologic examination in patients with probable Alzheimer's disease. *Archives of Neurology, 44*(9), 929-932.

Hurley, A.C., Volicer, B.J., Hanrahan, P.A., Houde, S., & Volicer, L. (1992). Assessment of discomfort in advanced Alzheimer patients. *Research in Nursing & Health, 15*(5), 369-377.

Hurley, M.V., Rees, J., & Newham, D.J. (1998). Quadriceps function, proprioceptive acuity and performance in healthy young, middle-aged and elderly subjects. *Age and Ageing, 27*(1), 55-62.

Hutchinson, S., Kobayashi, M., Horkan, C.M., Pascual-Leone, A., Alexander, M.P., Schlaug, G. (2002). Age-related differences in movement representation. *Neuroimage, 7(4)*, 1720-1728.

Hutchinson, M., & Fazzini, E. (1996). Cholinesterase inhibition in Parkinson's disease. *Journal of Neurology, Neurosurgery & Psychiatry, 61*(3), 324-325.

Ibach, B., Poljansky, S., Marienhagen, J., Sommer, M., Männer, P., & Hajak, G. (2004). Contrasting metabolic impairment in frontotemporal degeneration and early onset Alzheimer's disease. *NeuroImage, 23*(2), 739-743.

Imran, M.B., Kawashima, R., Awata, S., Sato, K., Kinomura, S., Ono, S., … Fukuda, H. (1999). Tc-99m HMPAO SPECT in the evaluation of Alzheimer's Disease: Correlation between neuro-psychiatric evaluation and CBF images. *Journal of Neurology, Neurosurgy & Psychiatry, 66*(2), 228-232.

Inzitari, M., Newman, A.B., Yaffe, K., Boudreau, R., de Rekeneire, N., Shorr, R., … Rosano, C. (2007). Gait speed predicts decline in attention and psychomotor speed in older adults: the health aging and body composition study. *Neuroepidemiology, 29*(3-4), 156-162.

Iseki, K., Hanakawa, T., Shinozaki, J., Nankaku, M., & Fukuyama, H. (2008). Neural mechanisms involved in mental imagery and observation of gait. *NeuroImage, 41*(3), 1021-1031.

Ishunina, T.A., & Swaab, D.F. (2002). Neurohypophyseal peptides in aging and Alzheimer's disease. *Ageing Research Reviews, 1*(3), 537–558.

Ivry, R.B., Keele, S.W., & Diener, H.C. (1988). Dissociation of the lateral and medial cerebellum in movement timing and movement execution. *Experimental Brain Research, 73*(1), 167-180.

Jack, C.R., Petersen, R.C., O'Brien, P.C., & Tangalos, E.G. (1992). MR-based hippocampal volumetry in the diagnosis of Alzheimer's disease. *Neurology, 42*(1), 183-188.

Jack, C.R., Petersen, R.C., Xu, Y.C., O'Brien, P.C., Smith, G.E., Ivnik, R.J., & Kokmen, E. (1999). Prediction of AD with MRI-based hippocampal volume in mild cognitive impairment. *Neurology, 52*(7), 1397-1403.

Jackson, G.R., Owsley, C., & McGwin, Jr., G., (1999). Aging and dark adaption. *Vision Research, 39* (23), 3975-3982.

Jackson, P.L., Lafleur, M.F., Malouin, F., Richards, C.L., & Doyon, J. (2003). Functional cerebral reorganization following motor sequence learning through mental practice with motor imagery. *NeuroImage, 20*(2), 1171-1180.

Jacobs, B.L., Heym, J., & Trulson, M.E. (1981). Behavioral and physiological correlates of brain serotonergic unit activity. *Journal de Physiologie, Paris, 77*(2-3), 431-436.

Jacobs, J., Bernhard, M., Delgado, A., & Strain, J.J. (1977). Screening for organic mental syndromes in the medically ill. *Annals of Internal Medicine, 86*(1), 40-46.

Jahn, K., Deutschländer, A., Stephan, T., Strupp, M., Wiesmann, M., & Brandt, T. (2004). Brain activation patterns during imagined stance and locomotion in functional magnetic resonance imaging. *NeuroImage, 22*(4), 1722-1731.

Jeka, J.J., & Lackner, J.R. (1994). Fingertip contact influences human postural control. *Experimental Brain Research, 100*(3), 495-502.

Jellinger, K.A. (2002). The pathology of ischemic-vascular dementia: An update. *Journal of the Neurological Sciences, 203*, 153-157.

Jellinger, K.A. (2003). alpha-synuclein pathology in Parkinson's and Alzheimer's disease brain: Incidence and topographic distribution – A pilot study. *Acta Neuropathologica, 106*(2), 191-201.

Jennings, C.R., & Jones, N.S. (2001). Presbyacusis. *The Journal of Laryngology & Otology, 115*(3), 171-178.

Jensen, M.P., Miller, L., & Fisher, L.D. (1998). Assessment of pain during medical procedures: a comparison of three scales. *Clinical Journal of Pain, 14*(4), 343-349.

Johnson, M.K., Mitchell, K.J., Raye, C.L., & Greene, E.J. (2004). An age-related deficit in prefrontal cortical function associated with refreshing information. *Psychological Science, 15*(2), 127-132.

Johnson, N.A., Jahng, G.-H., Weiner, M.W., Miller, B.L., Chui, H.C., Jagust, W.J., & Schuff, N. (2005). Pattern of cerebral hypoperfusion in Alzheimer disease and Mild Cognitive Impairment measured with arterial spin-labeling MR imaging: Initial experience. *Neuroradiology, 234*(3), 851-859.

Jones, S.L. (1991). Descending noradrenergic influences on pain. In: C.D. Barnes & O. Pompeiano (Eds.), *Progress in Brain Research, Vol. 88* (pp. 381-394).. Amsterdam: Elsevier Science.

Jonides, J,, Smith, E.E., Marshuetz, C., Koeppe, R.A., & Reuter-Lorenz, P.A. (1998). Inhibition in verbal working memory revealed by brain activation. *Proceedings of the National Academy of Science of the United States of America, 95*(14), 8410-8413.

Jueptner, M., Frith, C.D., Brooks, D.J., Frackowiak, R.S., & Passingham, R.E. (1997). Anatomy of motor learning. II. Subcortical structures and learning by trial and error. *Journal of Neurophysiology. 77*, 1325–1337.

Kaga, K., Nakamura, M., Takayama, Y., & Momose, H. (2004). A case of cortical deafness and anarthria. *Acta Otolaryngologica 124*(2), 202-205.

Kang, H.G., & Dingwell, J.B. (2008). Separating the effects of age and walking speed on gait variability. *Gait & Posture, 27*(4), 572–577.

Karlsen, K.H., Tandberg, E., Årsland, D., & Larsen, J.P. (2000). Health related quality of life in Parkinson's disease: A prospective longitudinal study. *Journal of Neurology, Neurosurgery and Psychiatry, 69*(5), 584-589.

Kashani, A., Lepicard, E., Poirel, O., Videau, C., David, J.P., Fallet-Bianco, C., … El Mestikawy, S. (2008). Loss of VGLUT1 and VGLUT2 in the prefrontal cortex is correlated with cognitive decline in Alzheimer disease. *Neurobiology of Aging, 29*(11), 1619-1630.

Kato, H., Yoshikawa, T., Oku, N., Imaizumi, M., Takasawa, M., Kimura, Y., … Hatazawa, J. (2008). Statistical parametric analysis of cerebral blood flow in vascular dementia with small-vessel disease using Tc-HMPAO SPECT. *Cerebrovasculair Diseases, 26*(5), 556-562.

Kato, M., Meguro, K., Sato, M., Shimada, Y., Yamazaki, H., Saito, H., & Yamadori, A. (2001). Ideomotor apraxia in patients with Alzheimer disease: Why do they use their body parts as objects? *Neuropsychiatry, Neuropsychology and Behavioral Neurology, 14*(1), 45-52.

Kayama, Y., & Koyama, Y. (1998). Brainstem neural mechanisms of sleep and wakefulness. *European Urology, 33*(Suppl. 3), 12-15.

Keane, W.L. (1994). The patient's perspective: The Alzheimer Association. *Alzheimer Disease and Associated Disorders, 8*(Suppl. 3), 151-155.

Keller, B.K., Morton, J.L., Thomas, V.S., & Potter, J.F. (1999). The effect of visual and hearing impairments on functional status. *Journal of the American Geriatric Society, 47*(11), 1319-1325.

Keller, J.N. (2005). Age-related neuropathology, cognitive decline, and Alzheimer's disease. *Ageing Research Reviews, 5*(1), 1-13.

Kelly, A.M., Hester, R., Murphy, K., Javitt, D.C., Foxe, J.J., & Garavan, H. (2004). Prefrontal-subcortical dissociations underlying inhibitory control revealed by event-related fMRI. *European Journal of Neuroscience, 19*(11), 3105-3112.

Kemppainen, N., Laine, M., Laakso, M.P., Kaasinen, V., Någren, K., Vahlberg, T., & Rinne, J.O. (2003). Hippocampal dopamine D2 receptors correlate with memory functions in Alzheimer's disease. *European Journal of Neuroscience, 18*(1), 149-154.

Kemppainen, N.M., Aalto, S., Wilson, I.A., Någren, K., Helin, S., Brück, A., ... Rinne, J.O. (2006). Voxel-based analysis of PET amyloid ligand [11C]PIB uptake in Alzheimer disease. *Neurology, 67* (9), 1575-1580.

Kennedy, P.J., & Shapiro, M.L. (2004). Retrieving memories via internal context requires the hippocampus. *Journal of Neuroscienc, 24*(31), 6979-6985.

Kenshalo, D.R. (1977). Age changes in touch, vibration, temperature, kinaesthesia and pain sensitivity. In: J.E. Birren & K.W. Schaie (Eds.), *Handbook of the Psychology of Aging* (pp. 562-579). New York: Van Nostrand.

Kenshalo, D.R. (1986). Somatesthetic sensitivity in young and elderly humans. *Journals of Gerontology, 41*(6), 732-742.

Keogh, J., Morrison, S., & Barrett, R. (2006). Age-related differences in inter-digit coupling during finger pinching. *European Journal of Applied Physiology, 97*(1), 76-88.

Kerns, R.D., Kassirer, M., & Otis, J. (2002). Pain in multiple sclerosis: A biopsychosocial perspective. *Journal of Rehabilitation Research and Development, 39*(2), 225-232.

Kerrouche, N., Herholz, K., Mielke, R., Holthoff, V., & Baron, J.C. (2006). (18)FDG PET in vascular dementia: Differentiation from Alzheimer's disease using voxel-based multivariate analysis. *Journal of Cerebral Blood Flow & Metabolism, 26*(9), 1213-1221.

Kersaitis, C., Halliday, G.M., & Kril, J.J. (2004). Regional and cellular pathology in frontotemporal dementia: Relationship to stage of disease in cases with and without Pick bodies. *Acta Neuropathologica, 108*(6), 515-523.

Kertesz, A., Blair, M., McMonagle, P., & Munoz, D.G. (2007). The diagnosis and course of frontotemporal dementia. *Alzheimer Disease & Associated Disorders, 21*(2), 155-163.

Kier, E.L., Staib, L.H., Davis, L.M., & Bronen, R.A. (2004). MR imaging of the temporal stem: Anatomic dissection tractography of the uncinate fasciculus, inferior occipitofrontal fasciculus, and Meyer's loop of the optic radiation. *American Journal of Neuroradiology, 25*(5), 677-691.

Kim, E.J., Rabinovici, G.D., Seeley, W.W., Halabi, C., Shu, H., Weiner, M.W., ... Rosen, H.J. (2007). Patterns of MRI atrophy in tau positive and ubiquitin positive frontotemporal lobar degeneration. *Journal of Neurology, Neurosurgery & Psychiatry, 78*(12), 1375-1378.

Kim, M.-A., Lee, H.S., Lee, B.Y., & Waterhouse, B.D. (2004). Reciprocal connections between subdivisions of the dorsal raphe and the nuclear core of the locus coeruleus in the rat. *Brain Research, 1026*(1), 56-67.

Kim, R.C., Ramachandran, T., Parisi, J.E., & Collins, G.H. (1981). Pallidonigral pigmentation and spheroid formation with multiple striatal lacunar infarcts. *Neurology, 31*(6), 774-777.

Kiosses, D.N., & Alexopoulos, G.S. (2005). IADL functions, cognitive deficits, and severity of depression - A preliminary study. *American Journal of Geriatric Psychiatry, 13*(3), 244-249.

Kirshenbaum, N., Riach, C.L., & Starkes, J.L. (2001). Non-linear development of postural control and strategy use in young children: A longitudinal study. *Experimental Brain Research, 140*(4), 420-431.

Kirshner, H.S., & Bakar, M. (1995). Syndromes of language dissolution in aging and dementia. *Comprehensive Therapy, 21*(9), 519-523.

Kivipelto, M., Ngandu, T., Fratiglioni, L., Viitanen, M., Kareholt, I., Winblad, B., ... Nissinen, A. (2005). Obesity and vascular risk factors at midlife and the risk of dementia and Alzheimer disease. *Archives of Neurology, 62*(10), 1556-1560.

Kluger, A., Gianutsos, J.G., Golomb, J., Ferris, S.H., George, A.E., Franssen, E., & Reisberg, B. (1997). Patterns of motor impairment in normal aging, mild cognitive decline, and early Alzheimer's disease. *Journals of Gerontology Series B-Psychological Sciences and Social Sciences, 52*(1), P28-P39.

Knopman, D.S., Parisi, J.E., Boeve, B.F., Cha, R.H., Apaydin, H., Salviati, A., & Rocca, W.A. (2003). Vascular dementia in a population-based autopsy study. *Archives of Neurology, 60*(4), 569-575.

Kobayashi, S., Tateno, M., Utsumi, K., Takahashi, A., Saitoh, M., Morii, H., ... Teraoka, M. (2008). Quantitative analysis of brain perfusion SPECT in Alzheimer's disease using a fully automated regional cerebral blood flow quantification software, 3DSRT. *Journal of the Neurological Sciences, 264*(1-2), 27-33.

Kocsis, B., & Vertes, R.P. (1992). Dorsal raphe neurons: Synchronous discharge with the theta rhythm of the hippocampus in the freely behaving rat. *Journal of Neurophysiology, 68*(4), 1463-1467.

Koistinaho, M., & Koistinaho, J. (2005). Interactions between Alzheimer's disease and cerebral ischemia – Focus on inflammation. *Brain Research Reviews, 48*(2), 240-250.

Kolanowski, A., Buettner, L., Litaker, M., & Yu, F. (2006). Factors that relate to activity engagement in nursing home residents. *American journal of Alzheimer's disease and other dementias, 21*(1), 15-22.

Koss, E., Weiffenbach, J.M., Haxby, J.V., & Friedland, R.P. (1988). Olfactory detection and identification performance are dissociated in early Alzheimer's disease. *Neurology, 38*(8), 1228-1232.

Kovach, C.R., Weissman, D.E., Griffie, J., Matson, S., & Muchka, S. (1999). Assessment and treatment of discomfort for people with late-stage dementia. *Journal of Pain and Symptom Management, 18* (6), 412-419.

Kovács, T., Cairns, N.J., & Lantos, P.L. (1999). Beta-amyloid deposition and neurofibrillary tangle formation in the olfactory olfactory bulb in ageing and Alzheimer's disease. *Neuropathology and Applied Neurobiology, 25*(6), 481-491.

Kovács, T. (2004). Mechanisms of olfactory dysfunction in aging and neurodegenerative disorders. *Ageing Research Reviews, 3*(2), 215-232.

Kramer, A.F., Bherer, L., Colcombe, S.J., Dong, W., & Greenough, W.T. (2004). Environmental influences on cognitive and brain plasticity during aging. *Journals of Gerontology Series A-Biological Sciences and Medical Sciences,59*(9), 940-957.

Kramer, A.F., Hahn, S., Cohen, N.J., Banich, M.T., McAuley, E., Harrison, C.R., ... Colcombe, A. (1999). Ageing, fitness and neurocognitive function. *Nature, 400*(6743), 418-419.

Krueger, C.E., Bird, A.C., Growdon, M.E., Jang, J.Y., Miller, B.L., & Kramer, J.H. (2009). Conflict monitoring in early frontotemporal dementia. *Neurology, 73*(5), 349-55.

Kuczynski, B., Jagust, W., Chui, H.C., & Reed. B. (2009). An inverse association of cardiovascular risk and frontal lobe glucose metabolism. *Neurology, 72*(8),738-743.

Kurlan, R., Richard, I.H., Papka, M., & Marshall, F. (2000). Movement disorders in Alzheimer's disease: more rigidity of definitions is needed. *Movement Disorders, 15*(1), 24-29.

Laakso, M.P., Frisoni, G.B., Kononen, M., Mikkonen, M., Beltramello, A., Geroldi, C., ... Aronen, H. J. (2000). Hippocampus and entorhinal cortex in frontotemporal dementia and Alzheimer's disease: a morphometric MRI study. *Biological Psychiatry, 47*(12), 1056-1063.

Lafleur, M.F., Jackson, P.L., Malouin, F., Richards, C.L., Evans, A.C., & Doyon, J. (2002). Motor learning produces parallel dynamic functional changes during the execution and imagination of sequential foot movements. *NeuroImage, 16*(1), 142-157.

Lalonde, R., & Badescu, R. (1995). Exploratory drive, frontal lobe function and adipsia in aging. *Gerontology, 41*(3), 134-144.

Larsson, M., Nilsson, L.-G., Olofsson, J.K., & Nordin, S. (2004). Demographic and cognitive predictors of cued odor identification: Evidence from a population-based study. *Chemical Senses, 29*(6), 547-554.

Lautenschlager, N.T., Cox, K.L., Flicker, L., Foster, J.K., van Bockxmeer, F.M., Xiao, J., … Almeida, O.P. (2008). Effect of physical activity on cognitive function in older adults at risk for Alzheimer disease: A randomized trial. *Journal of the American Medical Association, 300*(9), 1027-37.

Lazowski, D.A., Ecclestone, N.A., Myers, A.M., Paterson, D.H., Tudor-Locke, C., Fitzgerald, C., Cunningham, D.A. (1999). A randomized outcome evaluation of group exercise programs in long-term care institutions. *Journals of Gerontology Series A-Biological Sciences and Medical Sciences, 54*(12), M621-M628.

Lee, H.C.B., & Lyketsos, C.G. (2003). Depression in Alzheimer's disease: Heterogeneity and related issues. *Biological Psychiatry, 54*(3), 353-362.

Legoratti-Sanchez, M.O., Guevara-Guzman, R., & Solano-Flores, L.P. (1989). Electrophysiological evidences of bidirectional communication between the locus coeruleus and the suprachiasmatic nucleus. *Brain Research Bulletin, 23*(4-5), 283-288.

Leh, S.E., Ptito, A., Chakravarty, M.M., & Strafella, A.P. (2007). Fronto-striatal connections in the human brain: A probabilistic diffusion tractography study. *Neuroscience Letters, 419*(2), 113-118.

Leigland, L.A., Schulz, L.E., & Janowsky, J.S. (2004). Age related changes in emotional memory. *Neurobiology of Aging, 25*(8), 1117-1124.

Leiguarda, R.C., & Marsden, C.D. (2000). Limb apraxias: Higher-order disorders of sensorimotor integration. *Brain, 123*, 860-879.

Lezak, M. (1995). *Neuropsychological assessment.* New York: Oxford University Press.

Li, K.Z.H., & Lindenberger, U. (2002). Relations between aging sensory/sensorimotor and cognitive functions. *Neuroscience and Biobehavioral Reviews, 26*(7), 777-783.

Liao, D., Cooper, L., Cai, J., Toole, J.F., Bryan, N.R., Hutchinson, R.G., & Tyroler, H.A. (1996). Presence and severity of cerebral white matter lesions and hypertension, its treatment, and its control. *Stroke, 27*(12), 2262-2270.

Lijnen, H.R., & Collen, D. (1997). Endothelium in hemostasis and thrombosis. *Progress in Cardiovascular Diseases, 39*(4), 343-350.

Lindenberger, U., & Baltes, P.B. (1994). Sensory functioning and intelligence in old age: A strong connection. *Psychology and Aging, 9*(3), 339-355.

Lindenmuth, G.F., & Moose, B. (1990). Improving cognitive abilities of elderly Alzheimer's patients with intense exercise therapy. *American Journal of Alzheimer's Care and Related Disorders and Research, 5*, 31-33.

Lineweaver, T.T., Salmon, D.P., Bondi, M.W., Corey-Bloom, J. (2005). Differential effects of Alzheimer's disease and Huntington's disease on the performance of mental rotation. *Journal of the International Neuropsychological Society, 11*(1), 30-39.

Littbrand, H., Lundin-Olsson, L., Gustafson, Y., & Rosendahl, E. (2009). The effect of a high-intensity functional exercise program on activities of daily living: A randomized controlled trial in residential care facilities. *Journal of the American Geriatrics Society, 57*(10), 1741-1749.

Liu, Y., Ishida, Y., Shinoda, K., & Nakamura, S. (2003). Interaction between serotonergic and noradrenergic axons during axonal regeneration. *Experimental Neurology, 184*(1), 169-178.

Lolova, I., & Davidoff, M. (1991). Age-related changes in serotonin-immunoreactive neurons in the rat nucleus raphe dorsalis and nucleus centralis superior: A light microscope study. *Mechanisms of Ageing and Development, 62*(3), 279-289.

Lord, S.R., Clark, R.D., & Webster, I.W. (1991). Postural stability and associated physiological factors in a population of aged persons. *Journal of Gerontology, 46*(3), M69-M76.

Lorenz, J., Minoshima, S., & Casey, K.L. (2003). Keeping pain out of mind: The role of the dorsolateral prefrontal cortex in pain modulation. *Brain, 126*, 1079-1091.

Lucca, U., Tettamanti, M., Forloni, G., & Spagnoli, A. (1994). Nonsteroidal antiinflammatory drug use in Alzheimer's disease. *Biological Psychiatry, 36*(12), 854-856.

Luchsinger, J.A., & Mayeux, R. (2004). Cardiovascular risk factors and Alzheimer's disease. *Current atherosclerosis reports, 6*(4), 261-6.

Luciani, A., & Balducci, L. (2004). Multiple primary malignancies. *Seminars in Oncology, 31*(2), 264-273.

Luckhaus, C., Flüb, M.O., Wittsack, H.J., Grass-Kapanke, B., Jänner, M., Khalili-Amiri, R., ... Cohnen, M. (2008). Detection of changed regional cerebral blood flow in mild cognitive impairment and early Alzheimer's dementia by perfusion-weighted magnetic resonance imaging. *NeuroImage, 40*(2), 495-503.

Lüth, H.J., Ogunlade, V., Kuhla, B., Kientsch-Engel, R., Stahl, P., Webster, J., ... Münch, G. (2005). Age- and stage-dependent accumulation of advanced glycation end products in intracellular deposits in normal and Alzheimer's disease brains. *Cerebral Cortex, 15*(2), 211-220.

MacIntosh, C., Morley, J.E., & Chapman, I.M. (2000). The anorexia of aging. *Nutrition, 16*(10), 983-995..

Malouin, F., Richards, C.L., Jackson, P.L., Dumas, F., & Doyon, J. (2003). Brain activations during motor imagery of locomotor-related tasks: A PET study. *Human Brain Mapping, 19*(1), 47-62.

Manaye, K.F., McIntire, D.D., Mann, D.M., & German, D.C. (1995). Locus coeruleus cell loss in the aging human brain: A non-random process. *The Journal of Comparative Neurology, 358*(1), 79-87.

Manfredi, P.L., Breuer, B., Meier, D.E., & Libow, L. (2003a). Pain assessment in elderly patients with severe dementia. *Journal of Pain and Symptom Management, 25*(1), 48-52.

Manfredi, P.L., Breuer, B., Wallenstein, S., Stegmann, M., Bottomley, G., & Libow, L. (2003b) Opioid treatment for agitation in patients with advanced dementia. *International Journal of Geriatric Psychiatry, 18*(8), 700-705.

Manly, J.J., Bell-McGinty, S., Tang, M.X., Schupf, N., Stern, Y., & Mayeux, R. (2005). Implementing diagnostic criteria and estimating frequency of mild cognitive impairment in an urban community. *Archives of Neurology, 62*(11), 1739-1746.

Marcyniuk, B., Mann, D.M.A., & Yates, P.O. (1986). Loss of nerve cells from locus coeruleus in Alzheimer's disease is topographically arranged. *Neuroscience Letters, 64*(3), 247-252.

Marczinski, C.A., & Kertesz, A. (2005). Category and letter fluency in semantic dementia, primary progressive aphasia, and Alzheimer's disease. *Brain and Language, 97*(3), 258-265.

Markesbery, W.R, Schmitt, F.A., Kryscio, R.J., Davis, D.G, Smith, C.D., & Wekstein, D.R. (2006). Neuropathologic substrate of mild cognitive impairment. *Archives of Neurology, 63*(1), 38-46.

Marks, R., Quinney, H.A., & Wessel, J. (1993). Proprioceptive sensibility in women with normal and osteoarthritic knee joints. *Clinical Rheumatology, 12*(2), 170-175.

Marsh, R., Zhu, H., Schultz, R.T., Quackenbush, G., Royal, J., Skudlarski, P., & Peterson, B.S. (2006). A developmental fMRI study of self-regulatory control. *Human Brain Mapping, 27*(11), 848-863.

Martin, M., Clare, L., Altgassen, A.M., Cameron, M.H., & Zehnder, F. (2011). Cognition-based interventions for healthy older people and people with mild cognitive impairment. *Cochrane Database of Systematic Reviews, 1.*

Maruyama, M., Matsui, T., Tanji, H., Nemoto, M., Tomita, N., Ootsuki, M., & Sasaki, H. (2004). Cerebrospinal fluid tau protein and periventricular white matter lesions in patients with mild cognitive impairment. *Archives of Neurology, 61*(5), 716-720.

Marzinski, L.R. (1991). The tragedy of dementia: clinically assessing pain in the confused, nonverbal elderly. *Journal of the Gerontological Nursing, 17*(6), 25-28.

Massimo, L., Powers, C., Moore, P., Vesely, L., Avants, B., Gee, J., ... Grossman, M. (2009). Neuroanatomy of apathy and disinhibition in frontotemporal lobar degeneration. *Dementia and Geriatric Cognitive Disorders, 27*(1), 96-104.

Mattay, V.S., Fera, F., Tessitore, A., Hariri, A.R., Das, S., Callicott, J.H., & Weinberger, D.R. (2002). Neurophysiological correlates of age-related changes in human motor function. *Neurology, 58*(4), 630-635.

Mattson, M.P. (1998). Activities in cellular signalling pathways: A two-edged sword? *Neurobiology of Aging, 12*(4), 343-346.

Mazzeo, R.S., & Tanaka, H. (2001). Exercise prescription for the elderly. Current recommendations. *Sports Medicine, 31*(11), 809-818.

McCormick, W.C., Kukull, W.A., van Belle, G., Bowen, J.D., Teri, L., & Larson, E.B. (1994). Symptom patterns and comorbidity in the early stages of Alzheimer's disease. *Journal of the American Geriatrics Society, 42*(5), 517-521.

McEwen, B.S. (1991). When is stimulation too much of a good thing? *Neurobiology of Aging, 12*(4), 346-348.

McGeer, P.L., McGeer, E.G., Akiyama, H., Itagaki, S., Harrop, R., & Peppard, R. (1990). Neuronal degeneration and memory loss in Alzheimer's disease and aging. In: J. Eccles & O. Creutzfeldt (Eds.), *The Principles of design and operation of the brain* (pp. 410-431). Berlin: Springer-Verlag.

McGrath, P.A., Seifert, C.E., Speechley, K.N., Booth, J.C., Stitt, L., & Gibson, M.C. (1996). A new analogue scale for assessing children's pain: An initial validation study. *Pain, 64*(3), 435-443.

McKinney, M., & Jacksonville, M.C. (2005). Brain cholinergic vulnerability: Relevance to behavior and disease. *Biochemical Pharmacology, 70*(8), 1115-1124.

Mellet, E., Briscogne, S., Tzourio-Mazoyer, N., Ghaëm, O., Petit, L., Zago, L., ... Denis, M. (2000). Neural correlates of topographic mental exploration: the impact of route versus survey perspective learning. *NeuroImage, 12*(5), 588-600.

Meltzer, C.C., Zubieta, J.K., Brandt, J., Tune, L.E., Mayberg, H.S., & Frost, J.J. (1996). Regional hypometabolism in Alzheimer's disease as measured by positron emission tomography after correction for effects of partial volume averaging. *Neurology, 47*(2), 454-461.

Melzack, R. (1975). The McGill Pain Questionnaire: Major properties and scoring methods. *Pain, 1*(3), 275-295.

Mendez, M.F., Shapira, J.S., & Miller, B.L. (2005). Stereotypical movements and frontotemporal dementia. *Movement Disorders, 20*(6), 742-745.

Mergl, R., Tigges, P., Schröter, A., Möller, H.-J., & Hegerl, U. (1999). Digitized analysis of handwriting and drawing in healthy subjects: Methods, results and perspectives. *Journal of Neuroscience Methods, 90*(2), 157-169.

Mesulam, M. (2004). The cholinergic lesion of Alzheimer's disease: Pivotal factor or side show? *Learning & Memory, 11*(1), 43-49.

Mesulam, M., Shaw, P., Mash, D., & Weintraub, S. (2004). Cholinergic nucleus basalis tauopathy emerges early in the aging-MCI-AD continuum. *Annals of Neurology, 55*(6), 815-828.

Mesulam, M.-M. (1995). The cholinergic contribution to neuromodulation in the cerebral cortex. *Seminars in the Neurosciences, 7*(5), 297-307.

Metcalfe, J.S., McDowell, K., Chang, T.Y., Chen, L.C., Jeka, J.J., & Clark, J.E. (2005). Development of somatosensory-motor integration: An event-related analysis of infant posture in the first year of independent walking. *Developmental Psychobiology, 46*(1), 19-35.

Meyer, J.S., Rauch, G.M., Rauch, R.A., Haque, A., & Crawford, K. (2000). Cardiovascular and other risk factors for Alzheimer's disease and vascular dementia. *Vascular factors in Alzheimer's Disease, 903*, 411-423.

Middei, S., Geracitano, R., Caprioli, A., Mercuri, N., & Ammassari-Teule, M. (2004). Preserved fronto-striatal plasticity and enhanced procedural learning in a transgenic mouse model of Alzheimer's disease overexpressing mutant hAPPswe. *Learning & Memory, 11*(4), 447-452.

Mielke, R., & Heiss, W.D. (1998). Positron emission tomography for diagnosis of Alzheimer's disease and vascular dementia. *Journal of Neural Transmission, 53*(Suppl.), 237-250.

Mirakhur, A., Craig, D., Hart, D.J., McIlroy, S.P., & Passmore, A.P. (2004). Behavioural and psychological syndromes in Alzheimer's disease. *International Journal of Geriatric Psychiatry, 19*(11), 1035-1039.

Modrego, P.J., & Ferrández, J. (2004). Depression in patients with mild cognitive impairment increases the risk of developing dementia of Alzheimer type - A prospective cohort study. *Archives of Neurology, 61*(8), 1290-1293.

Mohr, C., Leyendecker, S., Mangels, I., Machner, B., Sander, T., & Helmchen, C. (2008). Central representation of cold-evoked pain relief in capsaicin induced pain: an event-related fMRI study. *Pain, 139*(2), 416-430.

Monsch, A.U., Bondi, M.W., Butters, N., Salmon, D.P., Katzman, R., & Thal, L.J. (1992). Comparisons of verbal fluency tasks in the detection of dementia of the Alzheimer type. *Archives of Neurology, 49*(12), 1253-8.

Morgan, D., Funk, M., Crossley, M., Basran, J., Kirk, A., & Dal Bello-Haas, V. (2007). The potential of gait analysis to contribute to differential diagnosis of early stage dementia: Current research and future directions. *Canadian Journal on Aging, 26*(1), 19-32.

Morgan, M., Bradshaw, J.L., Phillips, J.G., Mattingley, J.B., Iansek, R., & Bradshaw, J.A. (1994). Effects of hand and age upon abductive and adductive movements: A kinematic analysis. *Brain & Cognition, 25*(2), 194-206.

Mori, E. (2002). Impact of subcortical ischemic lesions on behavior and cognition. *Annals of the New York Academy of Sciences, 977*, 141-148.

Morley, J.E. (2001). Decreased food intake with aging. *Journal of Gerontology: Medical Sciences 56A* (Sp. Iss. 2), 81-88.

Morris, R., Petrides, M., & Pandya, D.N. (1999). Architecture and connections of retrosplenial area 30 in the rhesus monkey (Macaca mulatta). *European Journal of Neuroscience, 11*(7), 2506-2518.

Mortimer, J.A., & Graves, A.B. (1993). Education and other socioeconomic determinants of dementia and Alzheimer's disease. *Neurology, 43*(Suppl. 4), S39-S44.

Moulin, D.E. (1989). Pain in Multiple Sclerosis. *Neurologic Clinics, 7*(2), 321-331.

Mulder, T., Zijlstra, W., & Geurts, A. (2002). Assessment of motor recovery and decline. *Gait Posture, 16*(2), 198-210.

Mulder, Th., & Hochstenbach, J. (2003). Motor control and learning: Implications for neurological rehabilitation. In: R.J. Greenwood, T.M. McMillan, M.P. Barnes & C.D. Ward (Eds.). *Handbook of Neurological Rehabilitation* (pp. 143-157). New York: Psychology Press.

Muldowney, J.A.S. & Vaughan, D.N. (2002). Tissue-type plasminogen activator release: new frontiers in endothelial function. *Journal of the American College of Cardiology, 40*(5), 967-969.

Munoz, D.G., Dickson, D.W., Bergeron, C., Mackenzie, I.R., Delacourte, A., & Zhukareva, V. (2003). The neuropathology and biochemistry of frontotemporal dementia. *Annals of Neurology, 54* (Suppl. 5), S24-28.

Murphy, C,. Nordin, S., & Acosta, L. (1997). Odor learning, recall, and recognition memory in young and elderly adults. *Neuropsychology, 11*(1), 126-137.

Murphy, C. (1999). Loss of olfactory function in dementing disease. *Physiology & Behavior 66*(2), 177-182.

Murphy, C., Schubert, C.R., Cruickshanks, K.J., Klein, B.E.K., Klein, R., & Nondahl, D.M. (2002). Prevalence of olfactory impairment in older adults. *Journal of the American Medical Association, 288*(18), 2307-2312.

Musselman, K., & Brouwer, B. (2005). Gender-related differences in physical performance among seniors. *Journal of Aging & Physical Activity, 13*(3), 239–253.

Naggara, O., Oppenheim, C., Rieu, D., Raoux, N., Rodrigo, S., Dalla Barba, G., & Meder, J.F. (2006). Diffusion tensor imaging in early Alzheimer's disease. *Psychiatry Research-Neuroimaging, 146*(3), 243-249.

Nakamura, T., Ghilardi, M.F., Mentis, M., Dhawan, V., Fukuda, M., Hacking, A., ... Eidelberg, D. (2001). Functional networks in motor sequence learning: Abnormal topographies in Parkinson's disease. *Human Brain Mapping, 12*(1), 42-60.

Nakamura, T., Meguro, K., Yamazaki, H., Okuzumi, H., Tanaka, A., Horikawa, A., ... Sasaki, H. (1997). Postural and gait disturbance correlated with decreased frontal cerebral blood flow in Alzheimer disease. *Alzheimer Disease & Associated Disorders, 11*(3), 132-139.

Nardini, M., Jones, P., Bedford, R., & Braddick, O. (2008). Development of cue integration in human navigation. *Current Biology, 18*(9), 689-693.

Neary, D., Snowden, J., & Mann, D. (2005). *Frontotemporal dementia, 4*(11), 771-780.

Netz, Y., Axelrad, S., & Argov, E. (2007). Group physical activity for demented older adults – Feasibility and effectiveness. *Clinical Rehabilitation, 21*(11), 977-986.

Neufang, S., Specht, K., Hausmann, M., Güntürkün, O., Herpertz-Dahlmann, B., Fink, G.R., & Konrad, K. (2009). Sex differences and the impact of steroid hormones on the developing human brain. *Cerebral Cortex, 19*(2), 464–473.

Newson, R.S., & Kemps, E.B. (2005). General lifestyle activities as a predictor of current cognition and cognitive change in older adults: A cross-sectional and longitudinal examination. *Journals of Gerontology Series B-Psychological Sciences and Social Sciences, 60*(3), P113-P120.

Ng, K., Woo, J., Kwan, M., Sea, M., Wang, A., Lo, R., ... Henry, C.J.K. (2004). Effect of age and disease on taste perception. *Journal of Pain and Symptom Management, 28*(1), 28-34.

Nieoullon, A. (2002). Dopamine and the regulation of cognition and attention. *Progress in Neurobiology, 67*(1), 53-83.

Nowson, C.A., Worsley, A., Margerison, C., Jorna, M.K., Godfrey, S.J., & Booth, A. (2005). Blood pressure change with weight loss is affected by diet type in men. *American Journal of Clinical Nutrition, 81*(5), 983-989.

Nurmikko, T.J. (2000). Mechanisms of central pain. *Clinical Journal of Pain, 16*(2), S21-S25.

Nusbaum, N.J. (1999). Aging and sensory senescence. *Southern Medical Journal, 92*(3), 267-275.

Nyatsanza, S., Shetty, T., Gregory, C., Lough, S., Dawson, K., & Hodges, J.R. (2003). A study of stereotypic behaviours in Alzheimer's disease and frontal and temporal variant frontotemporal dementia. *Journal of Neurology, Neurosurgery & Psychiatry, 74*(10), 1398-1402.

Nyenhuis, D.L., Gorelick, P.B., Geenen, E.J., Smith, C.A., Gencheva, E., Freels, S., & deToledo-Morrell, L., (2004). The pattern of neuropsychological deficits in Vascular Cognitive Impairment-No Dementia (Vascular CIND). *Clinical Neuropsychologist, 18*(1), 41-49.

O'Brien, J., Perry, R., Barber, R., Gholkar, A., & Thomas, A. (2000). The association between white matter lesions on magnetic resonance imaging and noncognitive symptoms. *Annals of the New York Academy of Sciences, 903*, 482-489.

O'Keeffe, S.T., Kazeem, H., Pilpott, R.M., Playfer, J.R., Gosney, M., & Lye, M. (1996). Gait disturbance in Alzheimer's disease: A clinical study. *Age and Ageing 25*(4), 313-316.

O'Mahoney, D., Rowan, M., Feely, J., Walsh, J.B., & Coakley, D. (1994). Primary auditory pathway and reticular activating system dysfunction in Alzheimer's disease. *Neurology, 44*(11), 2089-2094.

Okumiya, K., Matsubayashi, K., Wada, T., Kimura, S., Doi, Y., & Ozawa, T. (1996). Effects of exercise on neurobehavioral function in community-dwelling older people more than 75 years of age. *Journal of the American Geriatrics Society, 44*(5), 569-572.

Olesen, P.J., Nagy, Z., Westerberg, H., & Klingberg, T. (2003). Combined analysis of DTI and fMRI data reveals a joint maturation of white and grey matter in a fronto-parietal network. *Cognitive Brain Research, 18*(1), 48-57.

Osawa, A., Maeshima, S., Shimamoto, Y., Maeshima, E., Sekiguchi, E., Kakishita, K., & Moriwaki, H. (2004). Relationship between cognitive function and regional cerebral blood flow in different types of dementia. *Disability & Rehabilitatio , 26*(12), 739-745.

Ostwald, S.K., Snowdon, D.A., Rysavy, D.M., Keenan, N.L., & Kane, R.L. (1989). Manual dexterity as a correlate of dependency in the elderly. *Journal of the American Geriatrics Society, 37*(10), 963-969.

Ouchi, Y., Yoshikawa, E., Futatsubashi, M., Okada, H., Torizuka, T., & Kaneko, M. (2004). Activation in the premotor cortex during mental calculation in patients with Alzheimer's disease: Relevance of reduction in posterior cingulate metabolism. *NeuroImage, 22*(1), 155-163.

Pacher, P., & Kecskemeti, V. (2004). Trends in the development of new antidepressants. Is there a light at the end of the tunnel? *Current Medicinal Chemistry, 11*(7), 925-943.

Palleschi, L., Vetta, F., DeGennaro, E., Idone, G., Sottosanti, G., Gianni, W., & Marigliano, V. (1996). Effect of aerobic training on the cognitive performance of elderly patients with senile dementia of Alzheimer type. *Archives of Gerontology and Geriatrics,* (Suppl. 5), 47-50.

Panegyres, P.K. (2004). The contribution of the study of neurodegenerative disorders to the understanding of human memory. *QJM an International Journal of Medicine, 97*(9), 555-567.

Pantoni, L., & Garcia, J.H. (1997). Pathogenesis of leukoaraiosis: A review. *Stroke, 28*(3), 652-659.

Parente, D.B., Gasparetto, E.L., da Cruz, L.C. Jr., Domingues, R.C., Baptista, A.C., Carvalho, A.C., & Domingues, R.C. (2008). Potential role of diffusion tensor MRI in the differential diagnosis of mild cognitive impairment and Alzheimer's disease. *American Journal of Roentgenology, 190*(5), 1369-1374.

Parkin, A.J., & Walter, B.M. (1992). Recollective experience, normal aging, and frontal dysfunction. *Psychology and Aging, 7*(2), 290-298.

Pascual, J., del Arco, C., González, A.M., Diaz, A. del Olmo, E., & Pazos, A. (1991). Regionally specific age-dependent decline in alpha2-adrenoceptoren: An autoradiographic study in human brain. *Neuroscience Letters, 133*(2), 279-283.

Paulesu, E., Frith, C.D., & Frackowiak, R.S.J. (1993). The neural correlates of verbal component of working memory. *Nature, 362*(6418), 342-345.

Pepeu, G., & Giovannini, M.G. (2004). Changes in acetylcholine extracellular levels during cognitive processes. *Learning & Memory, 11*(1), 21-27.

Pereira, F.S., Yassuda, M.S., Oliveira, A.M., & Forlenza, O.V. (2008). Executive dysfunction correlates with impaired functional status in older adults with varying degrees of cognitive impairment. *International Psychogeriatrics, 20*(6), 1104-1115.

Perry, R.J., & Hodges, J.R. (2000). Differentiating frontal and temporal variant frontotemporal dementia from Alzheimer's disease. *Neurology, 54*(12), 2277-2284.

Perry, R.J., Watson, P., & Hodges, J.R. (2000). The nature and staging of attention dysfunction in early (minimal and mild) Alzheimer's disease: Relationship to episodic and semantic memory impairment. *Neuropsychologia, 38*(3), 252-271.

Peters, J.M., Hummel, T., Kratzsch, T., Lötsch, J., Skarke, C., & Frölich, L. (2003). Olfactory function in mild cognitive impairment and Alzheimer's disease: An investigation using psychophysical and electrophysiological techniques. *American Journal of Psychiatry, 160*(11), 1995-2002.

Petrides, M., & Milner, B. (1982). Deficits on subject-ordered tasks after frontal and temporal-lobe lesions in man. *Neuropsychologia, 20*(3), 249-262.

Pettersson, A.F., Engardt, M., & Wahlund, L.O. (2002). Activity level and balance in subjects with mild Alzheimer's disease. *Dementia & Geriatric Cognitive Disorders, 13*(4), 213-216.

Pettersson, A.F., Olsson, E., & Wahlund, L.O. (2007). Effect of divided attention on gait in subjects with and without cognitive impairment. *Journal of Geriatric Psychiatry and Neurology, 20*(1), 58-62.

Piguet, O., Ridley, L., Grayson, D.A., Bennett, H.P., Creasy, H., Lye, T.C., & Broe, G.A, (2003). Are MRI white matter lesions clinically significant in the 'Old-Old'? Evidence from the Sydney older persons study. *Dementia and Geriatric Cognitive Disorders, 15*(3), 143-150.

Pihlajamaki, M., Tanila, H., Hänninen, T., Könönen, M., Laakso, M., Partanen, K., & Aronen, H.J. (2000). Verbal fluency activates the left medial temporal lobe: A functional magnetic resonance imaging study. *Annals of Neurology, 47*(4), 470-476.

Pizzolato, G., Chierichetti, F., Fabbri, M., Cagnin, A., Dam, M., Ferlin, G., & Battistin, L. (1996). Reduced striatal dopamine receptors in Alzheimer's disease: Single photon emission tomography study with the D2 tracer [123I]-IBZM. *Neurology, 47*(4), 1065-1068.

Podewils, L.J., Guallar, E., Kuller, L.H., Fried, L.P., Lopez, O.L., Carlson, M., & Lyketsos, C.G. (2005). Physical activity, APOE genotype, and dementia risk: Findings from the Cardiovascular Health Cognition Study. *American Journal of Epidemiology, 161*(7), 639-651.

Poehlman, E.T., Toth, M.J., Goran, M.I., Carpenter, W.H., Newhouse, P., & Rosen, C.J. (1997). Daily energy expenditure in free-living non-institutionalized Alzheimer's patients. *Neurology, 48*(4), 997-1002.

Pohjasvaara, T., Mantyla, R., Ylikoski, R., Kaste, M., & Erkinjuntti, T. (2003). Clinical features of MRI-defined subcortical vascular disease. *Alzheimer Disease & Associated Disorders, 17*(4), 236-242.

Pomeroy, V.M., Warren, C.M., Honeycombe, C., Briggs, R.S.J., Wilkinson, D.G., Pickering, R.M., & Steiner, A. (1999). Mobility and dementia: Is physiotherapy treatment during respite care effective? *International Journal of Geriatric Psychiatry, 14*(5), 389-397.

Porter, F.L., Malhotra, K.M., Wolf, C.M., Morris, J.C., Miller, J.P., & Smith, M.C. (1996). Dementia and response to pain in the elderly. *Pain, 68*(2-3), 413-421.

Potter, J.M., Evans, A.L., & Duncan, G. (1995). Gait speed and activities of daily living function in geriatric patients. *Archives of Physical Medicine and Rehabilitation, 76*(11), 997-999.

Powell, R.R. (1974). Psychological effects of exercise therapy upon institutionalized geriatric mental patients. *Journals of Gerontology, 29*(2), 157-161.

Prehogan, A., & Cohen, C.I. (2004). Motor dysfunction in dementias. *Geriatrics, 59*(11), 53-54.

Price, D. (2000). Psychological and neural mechanisms of the affective dimension of pain. *Science, 288*(5472), 1769-1772.

Pugh, K.G., & Lipsitz, L.A. (2002). The microvascular frontal subcortical syndrome of aging. *Neurobiology of Aging, 23*(3), 421-431.

Quick, M., & Sourkes, R.L. (1977). Central dopaminergic and serotonergic systems in the regulation of adrenal tyrosine hydroxylase. *Journal of Neurochemistry, 28*(1), 137-147.

Raadsheer, F.C., Tilders, F.J., & Swaab, D.F. (1994). Similar age related increase of vasopressin colocalization in paraventricular corticotropin-releasing hormone neurons in controls and Alzheimer patients. *Journal of Neuroendocrinology, 6*(2), 131-133.

Rabinovici, G.D., Seeley, W.W., Kim, E.J., Gorno-Tempini, M.L., Rascovsky, K., Pagliaro, T.A., ... Rosen, H.J. (2007). Distinct MRI atrophy patterns in autopsy-proven Alzheimer's disease and frontotemporal lobar degeneration. *American Journal of Alzheimer's Disease & Other Dementias, 22*(6), 474-488.

Rahman, N., Thomas, J.J., & Rice, M.S. (2002). The relationship between hand strength and the forces used to access containers by well elderly persons. *American Journal of Occupational Therapy, 56*(1), 78-85.

Rainero, I., Vighetti, S., Bergamasco, B., Pinessi, L., & Benedetti, F. (2000). Autonomic responses and pain perception in Alzheimer's disease. *European Journal of Pain, 4*(3), 267-274.

Ranganathan, V.K., Siemionow, V., Sahgal, V., & Yue, G.H. (2001a). Effects of aging on hand function. *Journal of the American Geriatrics Society, 49*(11), 1478-1484.

Ranganathan, V.K., Siemionow, V., Sahgal, V., Liu, J.Z., & Yue, G.H. (2001b). Skilled finger movements exercise improves hand function. *Journals of Gerontology Series A-Biological Sciences and Medical Sciences, 56*(8), M518-522.

Rao, G. (2001). Insulin resistance syndrome. *American Family Physician, 63*(6), 1159-1163.

Rao, S.M., Bobholz, J.A., Hammeke, T.A., Rosen, A.C., Woodley, S.J., Cunningham, J.M., ... Binder, J.R. (1997). Functional MRI evidence for subcortical participation in conceptual reasoning skills. *Neuroreport, 8*(8), 1987-1993.

Rascovsky, K., Salmon, D.P., Ho, G.J., Galasko, D., Peavy, G.M., Hansen, L.A., & Thal, L.J. (2002). Cognitive profiles differ in autopsy-confirmed frontotemporal dementia and AD. *Neurology, 58* (12), 1801-1808.

Raz, N., Lindenberger, U., Rodrique, K.M., Kennedy, K.M., Head, D., Williamson, A., & Acker, J.D. (2005). Regional brain changes in aging healthy adults: General trends, individual differences and modifiers. *Cerebral Cortex, 15*(11), 1676-1689.

Raz, N., Rodrique, K.M., Head, D., Kennedy, K.M., & Acker, J.D. (2004). Differential aging of the medial temporal lobe. *Neurology, 62*(3), 433-438.

Raz, N., Rodrique, K.M., Kennedy, K.M., Head, D., Gunning-Dixon, F., & Acker, J.D.. (2003). Differential aging of the human striatum: Longitudinal evidence. *American Journal Neuroradiology, 24* (9), 1849-1856.

Raz, N., Torres, I.J., & Spencer, W.D. (1993). Pathoclysis in aging human cerebral cortex: Evidence from in vivo MRI morphometry. *Psychobiology, 21*(2), 151-160.

Reed, B.R., Eberling, J.L., Mungas, D., Weiner, M., Kramer, J.H., & Jagust, W.J. (2004). Effects of white matter lesions and lacunes on cortical function. *Archives of Neurology, 61*(10), 1545-1550.

Reeves, S., Bench, C., & Howard, R. (2002). Ageing and the nigrostriatal dopaminergic system. *International Journal of Geriatric Psychiatry, 17*(4), 359-370.

Regeur, L., Jensen, G.B., Pakkenberg, H, Evans, S.M., & Pakkeberg, B. (1994). No global neocortical nerve cell loss in brains from patients with senile dementia of Alzheimer's type. *Neurobiology, 15* (3), 347-352.

Reisberg, B., Franssen, E.H., Souren, L.E., Auer, S.R., Akram, I., & Kenowsky, S. (2002). Evidence and mechanisms of retrogenesis in Alzheimer's and other dementias: Management and treatment import. *American Journal of Alzheimer's Disease & Other Dementias. 17*(4), 202–212.

Rémy, F., Mirrashed, F., Campbell, B., & Richter, W. (2005). Verbal episodic memory impairment in Alzheimer's disease: A combined structural and functional MRI study. *NeuroImage, 25*(1), 253-266.

Reusch, J.E.B. (2002). Current concepts in insulin resistance, type 2 diabetes mellitus, and the metabolic syndrome. *American Journal of Cardiology, 90*(5A), 19G-26G.

Reuter-Lorenz, P.A., & Lustig, C. (2005). Brain aging: Reorganizing discoveries about the aging mind. *Current Opinion in Neurobiology, 15*(2), 245-251.

Richard, I.H., Justus, A.W., Greig, N.H., Marshall, F., & Kurlan, R. (2002). Worsening of motor function and mood in a patient with Parkinson's disease after pharmacologic challenge with oral rivastigmine. *Clinical Neuropharmacology, 25*(6), 296-9.

Richards, B.A., Chertkow, H., Singh, V., Robillard, A., Massoud, F., Evans, A.C., & Kabani, N.J. (2009). Patterns of cortical thinning in Alzheimer's disease and frontotemporal dementia. *Neurobiology of Aging 30*(10), 1626-1636.

Richards, M., Stern, Y., Marder, K., Cote, L., & Mayeux, R. (1993). Persistent extrapyramidal signs are a risk factor for dementia in aging. *Neurology, 43*(4), A276-A277.

Richardson, R.T,, & DeLong, M.R. (1988). A reappraisal of the functions of the nucleus basalis of Meynert. *Trends in Neuroscience, 11*(6), 264-267.

Ridler, K., Veijola, J.M., Tanskanen, P., Miettunen, J., Chitnis, X., Suckling, J., ... Bullmore, E.T. (2006). Fronto-cerebellar systems are associated with infant motor and adult executive functions in healthy adults but not in schizophrenia. *Proceedings of the National Academy of Sciences of the United States of America, 103*(42), 15651-15656.

Riecker, A., Mathiak, K., Wildgruber, D., Erb, M., Hertrich, I., Grodd, W., & Ackermann, H. (2005). fMRI reveals two distinct cerebral networks subserving speech motor control. *Neurology, 64*(4), 700-706.

Riggs, J.E. (1996). Differential survival, natural selection, and the manifestation of senescence. *Mechanisms of Ageing and Development, 87*(2), 91-98.

Rinne, J.O., Laine, M., Kaasinen, V., Norvasuo-Heila, M.K., Nagren, K., & Helenius, H. (2002). Striatal dopamine transporter and extrapyramidal symptoms in frontotemporal dementia. *Neurology, 58*(10), 1489-1493.

Rival, C., Ceyte, H., & Olivier, I. (2005). Developmental changes of static standing balance in children. *Neuroscience Letters, 376*(2), 133-136.

Robbins, T.W., & Everitt, B.J. (1995). Arousal systems and attention. In: M.S. Gazzaniga et al. (Eds.), *The Cognitive Neurosciences* (pp. 703-720). Cambridge: Mit Press.

Roberson, E.D., Hesse, J.H., Rose, B.A., Slama, H., Johnson, J.K., Yaffe, K., & Miller, B.L. (2005). Frontotemporal dementia progresses to death faster than Alzheimer disease. *Neurology, 65*(5), 719-725.

Rocca, M.A., Matthews, P.M., Caputo, D., Ghezzi, A., Falini, A., Scotti, G., ... Filippi, M. (2002). Evidence for widespread movement-associated functional MRI changes in patients with PPMS. *Neurology, 58*(6), 866-872.

Rolland, Y., Rival, L., Pillard, F., Lafont, C.H., Riviere, D., Albarede, J.-L., & Vellas, B. (2000). Feasibility of regular physical exercise for patients with moderate to severe Alzheimer disease. *The Journal of Nutrion, Health & Aging, 4*(2), 109-113.

Rolls, E.T. (1999). Spatial view cells and the representation of place in the primate hippocampus. *Hippocampus, 9*(4), 467-480.

Román, G.C. (2004). Vascular dementia: Advances in nosology, diagnosis, treatment and prevention. *Panminerva Medica, 46*(4), 207-215.

Román, G.C. (2005). Cholinergic dysfunction in vascular dementia. *Current Psychiatry Reports, 7*(1), 18-26.

Román, G.C., & Kalaria, R.N. (2005). Vascular determinants of cholinergic deficits in Alzheimer disease and vascular dementia. *Neurobiology of Aging, 27*(12), 1769-1785.

Román, G.C., & Kalaria, R.N. (2006). Vascular determinants of cholinergic deficits in Alzheimer disease and vascular dementia. *Neurobiology of Aging, 27*(12), 1769-1785.

Román, G.C., Erkinjuntti, T., Wallin, A., Pantoni, L., & Chui, H.C. (2002). Subcortical ischaemic vascular dementia. *Lancet Neurology, 1*(7), 426-436.

Rombouts, S.A., van Swieten, J.C., Pijnenburg, Y.A., Goekoop, R., Barkhof, F., & Scheltens, P. (2003). Loss of frontal fMRI activation in early frontotemporal dementia compared to early AD. *Neurology, 60*(12), 1904-1908.

Roncesvalles, M.N., Woollacott, M.H., & Jensen, J.L. (2000). The development of compensatory stepping skills in children. *Journal of Motor Behavior, 32*(1), 100-111.

Rosano, C., Simonsick, E.M., Harris, T.B., Kritchevsky, S.B., Brach, J., Visser, M., Yaffe, K., & Newman, A.B. (2005). Association between physical and cognitive function in healthy elderly: the health, aging and body composition study. *Neuroepidemiology, 24*(1-2), 8-14

Rosano, C., Aizenstein, H.J., Studenski, S., & Newman, A.B. (2007). A regions-of-interest volumetric analysis of mobility limitations in community-dwelling older adults. *Journals of Gerontology Series A-Biological Sciences and Medical Sciences, 62*(9), 1048-1055.

Rose, S.E., Chen, F., Chalk, J.B., Zelaya, F.O., Strugnell, W.E., Benson, M., ... Doddrell, D.M. (2000). Loss of connectivity in Alzheimer's disease: An evaluation of white matter tract integrity with colour coded MR diffusion tensor imaging. *Journal of Neurology, Neurosurgery & Psychiatry, 69*(4), 528-530.

Rosen, H.J., Allison, S.C., Schauer, G.F., Gorno-Tempini, M.-L., Weiner, M.W., & Miller, B.L. (2005). Neuroanatomical correlates of behavioural disorders in dementia. *Brain, 128*, 2612-2625.

Rosen, H.J., Hartikainen, K.M., Jagust, W., Kramer, J.H., Reed, B.R., Cummings, J.L., & Miller, B.L. (2002). Utility of clinical criteria in differentiating frontotemporal lobar degeneration (FTLD) from AD. *Neurology, 58*(11), 1608-1615.

Rosén, I., Gustafson, L., & Risberg, J. (1993). Multichannel EEG frequency analysis and somatosensory-evoked potentials in patients with different types of organic dementia. *Dementia, 4*(1), 43-49.

Rosengarten, B., Aldinger, C., Spiler, A., & Kaps, M. (2003). Neurovascular coupling remains unaffected during normal aging. *Journal of Neuroimaging, 13*(1), 43-47.

Roses, A.D. (1994). Apolipoprotein E affects the rate of Alzheimer disease expression: B-Amyloid burden is a secondary consequence dependent on APOE genotype and duration of disease. *Journal of Neuropathology and Experimental Neurology, 53*(5), 429-437.

Rosser, A., & Hodges, J.R. (1994). Initial letter and semantic category fluency in Alzheimer's disease, Huntington's disease, and progressive supranuclear palsy. *Journal of Neurology, 57*(11), 1389-1394.

Rossi, S., Miniussi, C., Pasqualetti, P., Babiloni, C., Rossini, P.M., & Cappa, S.F. (2004). Age-related functional changes of prefrontal cortex in long-term memory: A repetitive transcranial magnetic stimulation study. *The Journal of Neuroscience, 24*(36), 7939-7944.

Rossini, P.M., Filippi, M.M., & Vernieri, F. (1998). Neurophysiology of sensorimotor integration in Parkinson's disease. *Clinical Neuroscience, 5*(2), 121-30.

Rovio, S., Kåreholt, I., Helkala, E.-L., Viitanen, M., Winblad, B., Tuomilehto, J., ... Kivipelto, M. (2005). Leisure-time physical activity at midlife and the risk of dementia and Alzheimer's disease. *Lancet Neurology, 4*(11), 705-711.

Rüb, U., Del Tredici, K., Schultz, C., Ghebremedhin, E., de Vos, R.A., Jansen Steur, E., & Braak, H. (2002). Parkinson's disease: The thalamic components of the limbic loop are severely impaired by α-synuclein immunopositive inclusion body pathology. *Neurobiology of Aging, 23*(2), 245-254.

Rubia, K., Overmeyer, S., Taylor, E., Brammer, M., Williams, S.C., Simmons, A., ... Bullmore, E.T. (2000). Functional frontalisation with age: Mapping neurodevelopmental trajectories with fMRI. *Neuroscience & Biobehavioral Reviews, 24*(1), 13-19.

Rubia, K., Smith, A.B., Taylor, E., & Brammer, M. (2007). Linear age-correlated functional development of right inferior fronto-striato-cerebellar networks during response inhibition and anterior cingulate during error-related processes. *Human Brain Mapping, 28*(11), 1163–1177.

Rubia, K., Smith, A.B., Woolley, J., Nosarti, C., Heyman, I., Taylor, E., & Brammer, M. (2006). Progressive increase of frontostriatal brain activation from childhood to adulthood during event-related tasks of cognitive control. *Human Brain Mapping. 27*(12), 973-993.

Rushworth, M.F., Walton, M.E., Kennerley, S.W., & Bannerman, D.M. (2004). Action sets and decisions in the medial frontal cortex. *Trends in Cognitive Science, 8*(9), 410-417.

Sachdev, P.S., Wen, W., Christensen, H., & Form, A.F. (2005). White matter hyperintensities are related to physical disability and poor motor function. *Journal of Neurology, Neurosurgery & Psychiatry, 76*(3), 362-367.

Sadek, J.R., Johnson, S.A., White, D.A., Salmon, D.P., Taylor, K.I., DeLaPena, J.H., & Grant, I. (2004). Retrograde amnesia in dementia: Comparison of HIV-associated dementia, Alzheimer's disease, and Huntington's disease. *Neuropsychology, 18*(4), 692-699.

Sahyoun, C., Floyer-Lea, A., Johansen-Berg, H., & Matthews, P.M. (2004). Towards an understanding of gait control: brain activation during the anticipation, preparation and execution of foot movements. *NeuroImage, 21*(2), 568-575.

Salat, D.H., Buckner, R.L., Snyder, A.Z., Greve, D.N., Desikan, R.S.R., Busa, E., & Fischl, B. (2004). Thinning of the cerebral cortex in aging. *Cerebral Cortex, 14*(7), 721-730.

Salat, D.H., Kaye, J.A., & Janowsky, J.S. (2001). Selective preservation and degeneration within the prefrontal cortex in aging and Alzheimer's disease. *Archives of Neurology, 58*(9), 1403-1408.

Salthouse, T.A. (1996). The processing-speed theory of adult age differences in cognition. *Psychological Review, 103*(3), 403-428.

Santana-Sosa, E., Barriopedro, M.I., López-Mojares, M., Pérez, M., & Lucia, A. (2008). Exercise training is beneficial for Alzheimer's patients. *International Journal of Sports Medicine, 29*(10), 845-850.

Sapolsky, R.M. (1991). Energetics and neuron death: Hibernating bears or starving refugees? *Neurobiology of Aging, 12*(4), 348 349.

Sargolini, F., Fyhn, M., Hafting, T., McNaughton, B.L., Witter, M.P., Moser, M.B., & Moser, E.I. (2006). Conjunctive representation of position, direction, and velocity in entorhinal cortex. *Science, 312*(5774), 758-762.

Sato, A., Sato, Y., & Uchida, S. (2002). Regulation of cerebral cortical blood flow by the basal forebrain cholinergic fibers and aging. *Autonomic Neuroscience: Basic and Clinical, 96*(1), 13-19.

Sauvage, M., & Steckler, T. (2001). Detection of corticotropin-releasing hormone receptor 1 immunoreactivity in cholinergic, dopaminergic and noradrenergic neurons of the murine basal forebrain and brainstem nuclei - Potential for arousal and attention. *Neuroscience, 104*(3), 643-652.

Sawamoto, N., Honda, M., Hanakawa, T., Aso, T., Inoue, M., Toyoda, H., ... Shibasaki, H. (2007). Cognitive slowing in Parkinson's Disease is accompanied by hypofunctioning of the striatum. *Neurology, 68*(13), 1062-1068.

Scafetta, N., Marchi, D., & West, B.J. (2009). Understanding the complexity of human gait dynamics. *Chaos, 19*(2), 026108.

Schablowski-Trautmann, M., & Gerner, H.J. (2006). State-space analysis of joint angle kinematics in normal treadmill walking. *Biomedizinische Technik, 51*(5-6), 294-298.

Scheff, S.W., Price, D.A., Schmitt, F.A., & Mufson, E.J. (2005). Hippocampal synaptic loss in early Alzheimer's disease and mild cognitive impairment. *Neurobiology of Aging, 27*(10), 1372-1384.

Scheltens, P., & Kittner, B. (2000). Preliminary results from an MRI/CT-based database for vascular dementia and Alzheimer's disease. *Annals New York Academy of Sciences, 903*, 542-546.

Schenkman, M., Wei Zhu, C., Cutson, T.M., & Whetten-Goldstein, K. (2001). Longitudinal evaluation of economic and physical impact of Parkinson's disease. *Parkinsonism & Related Disorders, 8* (1), 41-50.

Scherder, E., Bouma, A., Slaets, J., Ooms, M., Ribbe, M., Blok, A., & Sergeant, J. (2001). Repeated pain assessment in Alzheimer's disease. *Dementia and Geriatric Cognitive Disorders, 12*(6), 400-407.

Scherder, E., Eggermont, L., Swaab, D., van Heuvelen, M., Kamsma, Y., de Greef, M., ... Mulder, T. (2007). Gait in ageing and associated dementias: Its relationship with cognition. *Neuroscience & Biobehavioral Reviews, 31*(4), 485-497.

Scherder, E.J.A., & Bouma, A. (2000). Visual analogue scales for pain assessment in Alzheimer's disease. *Gerontology, 46*(1), 47-53.

Scherder, E.J.A., Sergeant, J.A., & Swaab, D.F. (2003a). Pain processing in dementia and its relation to neuropathology. *Lancet Neurology, 2*(11), 677-686.

Scherder, E.J.A., Slaets, J., Deijen, J.-B., Gorter, Y., Ooms, M.E., Ribbe, ... Sergeant, J.A. (2003b). Pain assessment in patients with possible vascular dementia. *Psychiatry, 66*(2), 133-145.

Scherder, E.J.A., van Paasschen, J., Deijen, J.B., van der Knokke, S., Orlebeke, J.F.K., Burgers, I., ... Sergeant, J.A. (2005). Physical activity and executive functions in the elderly with mild cognitive impairment. *Aging & Mental Health, 9*(3), 272-280.

Schiffman, S.S., Clark, C.M., & Warwick, Z.S. (1990). Gustatory and olfactory dysfunction in dementia – Not specific to Alzheimer's disease. *Neurobiology of Aging, 11*(6), 597-600.

Schiffmann, S.S. (1997). Taste and smell losses in normal aging and disease. *Journal of the American Medical Association, 278*(16), 1357-1362.

Schiffmann, S.S. (2000). Intensification of sensory properties of foods for the elderly. *Journal of Nutrition, 130*(4), 927S-930S.

Schilke, J.M. (1991). Slowing the aging process with physical activity. *Journal of Gerontological Nursing, 17*(6), 4-8.

Schini-Kerth, V.B. (1999). Dual effects of insulin-like growth factor-I on the constitutive and inducible nitric oxide (NO) synthase-dependent formation of NO in vascular cells. *Journal of Endocrinological Investigation, 22*(Suppl. 5), 82-88.

Schmader, K.E., Hanlon, J.T., Fillen-Baum, G.G., Huber, M., Pieper, C., & Horner, R. (1998). Medication use patterns among demented, cognitively impaired and cognitively intact community-dwelling elderly people. *Age and Ageing, 27*(4), 493-501.

Schmahmann, J.D., & Leifer, D. (1992). Parietal pseudothalamic pain syndrome. *Archives of Neurology, 49*(10), 1032–1037.

Schmahmann, J.D., Pandya, D.N., Wang, R., Dai, G., D'Arceuil, H.E., de Crespigny, A.J., & Wedeen, V.J. (2007). Association fibre pathways of the brain: Parallel observations from diffusion spectrum imaging and autoradiography. *Brain, 130*, 630-653.

Schmidt, R., Schmidt, H., & Fazekas, F. (2000). Vascular risk factors in dementia. *Journal of Neurology, 247*(2), 81-87.

Schmidt, R.F., & Wahren, L.K. (1990). Multiunit neural responses to strong finger pulp vibration. II. Comparison with tactile sensory thresholds. *Acta Psychologica Scandinavica, 140*(1), 11-16.

Schott, G.D. (1985). Pain in Parkinson's disease. *Pain, 22*(4), 407-411.

Schröter, A., Mergl, R., Bürger, K., Hampel, H., Möller, H.-J., & Hegerl, U. (2003). Kinematic analysis of handwriting movements in patients with Alzheimer's Disease, mild cognitive impairment, depression and healthy subjects. *Dementia & Geriatric Cognitive Disorders, 15*(3), 132-142.

Schubotz, R.I., & von Cramon, D.Y. (2001). Interval and ordinal properties of sequences are associated with distinct premotor areas. *Cerebral Cortex, 11*(3), 210-222.

Seeley, W.W., Bauer, A.M., Miller, B.L., Gorno-Tempini, M.L., Kramer, J.H., Weiner, M., & Rosen, H.J. (2005). The natural history of temporal variant frontotemporal dementia. *Neurology, 64*(8), 1384-1390.

Segalowitz, S.J., & Davies, P.L. (2004). Charting the maturation of the frontal lobe: An electrophysiological strategy. *Brain & Cognition, 55*(1), 116-133.

Seidman, M.D., Ahmad, N., & Bai, U. (2002). Molecular mechanisms of age-related hearing loss. *Ageing Research Reviews, 1*(3), 331-343.

Seo, D., & Patrick, C.J. (2008). Role of serotonin and dopamine system interactions in the neurobiology of impulsive aggression and its comorbidity with other clinical disorders. *Aggression and Violent Behavior,13*(5), 383-395.

Sewards, T.V., & Sewards, M.A. (2002). The medial pain system: Neural representations of the motivational aspect of pain. *Brain Research Bulletin, 59*(3), 163-180.

Sharma, A.M., & Chetty, V.T. (2005). Obesity, hypertension and insulin resistance. *Acta Diabetolica, 42*(Suppl. 1), S3-S8.

Sheridan, P.L., & Hausdorff, J.M. (2007). The role of higher-level cognitive function in gait: Executive dysfunction contributes to fall risk in Alzheimer's disease. *Dementia & Geriatric Cognitive Disorders, 24*(2), 125-137.

Sheridan, P.L., Solomont, J., Kowall, N., & Hausdorff, J.M. (2003). Influence of executive functions on locomotor function: Divided attention increases gait variability in Alzheimer's disease. *Journal of the American Geriatrics Society, 51*(11), 1633-1637.

Shibasaki, H., & Kuroiwa, Y. (1974). Painful tonic seizure in multiple sclerosis. *Archives of Neurology, 30*(1), 47-51.

Shiffman, L.M. (1992). Effects of aging on adult hand function. *American Journal of Occupational Therapy, 46*(9), 785-792.

Shiflett, M.W., Tomaszycki, M.L., Rankin, A.Z., & de Voogd, T.J. (2004). Long-term memory for spatial locations in a food-storing bird (Poecile atricapilla) requires activation of NMDA receptors in the hippocampal formation during learning. *Behavioral Neuroscience 118*(1), 121-130.

Shim, J.K., Lay, B.S., Zatsiorsky, V.M., & Latash, M.L. (2004). Age-related changes in finger coordination in static prehension tasks. *Journal of Applied Physiology, 97*(1), 213-224.

Shim, Y.S., Yang, D.W., Kim, B.S., Shon, Y.M., & Chung, Y.A. (2006). Comparison of regional cerebral blood flow in two subsets of subcortical ischemic vascular dementia: Statistical parametric mapping analysis of SPECT. *Journal of the Neurological Sciences, 250*(1-2), 85-91.

Siever, L.J. (2008). Neurobiology of aggression and violence. *American Journal of Psychiatry, 165*(4), 429-442.

Silverman, S.E., Tran, D.B., Zimmerman, K.M., & Feldon, S.E. (1994). Dissociation between the detection and perception of motion in Alzheimer's disease. *Neurology, 44*(10), 1814-1818.

Sinha, U.K., Hollen, K.M., Rodriguez, R., & Miller, C.A. (1993). Auditory system degeneration in Alzheimer's disease. *Neurology, 43*(4), 779-785.

Sinha, U.K., Saadat, D., Linthicum, F.H., Hollen, K.M., & Miller, C.A. (1996). Temporal bone findings in Alzheimer's disease. *Laryngoscope, 106*(1), 1-5.

Sitzer, D.I., Twamley, E.W., & Jeste, D.V. (2006). Cognitive training in Alzheimer's disease: a meta-analysis of the literature. *Acta Psychiatrica Scandinavica, 114*(2), 75–90.

Skinner, H.B., Wyatt, M.P., Hodgdon, J.A., Conard, D.W., & Barrack, R.L. (1986). Effect of fatigue on joint position sense of the knee. *Journal of Orthopeadic Research, 4*(1), 112-118.

Skoog, I. (2004). Psychiatric epidemiology of old age: the H70 study – the NAPE Lecture 2003. *Acta Psychiatrica Scandinavica, 109*(1), 4-18.

Slavin, M.J., Phillips, J.G., Bradshaw, J.L., Hall, K.A., & Presnell, I. (1999). Consistency of handwriting movements in dementia of the Alzheimer's type: A comparison with Huntington's and Parkinson's diseases. *Journal of the International Neuropsychological Society, 5*(1), 20-25.

Small, S.A., Stern, Y., Tang, M., & Mayeux, R. (1999). Selective decline in memory function among healthy elderly. *Neurology, 52*(7), 1392-1396.

Smith, C.D., Umberger, G.H., Manning, E.L., Slevin, J.T., Wekstein, D.R., Schmitt, F.A., … Gash, D.M. (1999). Critical decline in fine motor hand movements in human aging. Neurology, 53(7), 1458-1461.

Smith, C.D., Walton, A., Loveland, A.D., Umberger, G.H., Kryscio, R.J., & Gash, D.M. (2005). Memories that last in old age: Motor skill learning and memory preservation. *Neurobiology of Aging 26* (6), 883-890.

Smith, I.M., & Bryson, S.E. (2007). Gesture imitation in autism: II. Symbolic gestures and pantomimed object use. *Cognitive Neuropsychology. 24*(7), 679-700.

Smith, M.A. (1996). Hippocampal vulnerability to stress and aging: Possible role of neurotrophic factors. *Behavioural Brain Research, 78*(1), 25-36.

Snijders, A.H., Nijkrake, M.J., Bakker, M., Munneke, M., Wind, C., & Bloem, B.R. (2008). Clinimetrics of freezing of gait. *Movement Disorders, 23*(Suppl. 2), S468-S474.

Snook, L., Paulson, L.A., Roy, D., Phillips, L., & Beaulieu, C. (2005). Diffusion tensor imaging of neurodevelopment in children and young adults. *Neuroimage, 26*(4), 1164-1173.

Snow, A.L., Weber, J.B., O'Malley, K.J., Cody, M., Beck, C., Bruera, E., … Kunik, M.E. (2004). NOPPAIN: A nursing assistant-administered pain assessment instrument for use in dementia. *Dementia and Geriatric Cognitive Disorders, 17*(3), 240-246.

Sofroniew, M.V. (1991). Can activity modulate the susceptibility of neurons to degeneration? *Neurobiology of Aging, 12*(4), 351-352.

Solaro, C., Lunardi, G.L., & Mancardi, G.L. (2003). Pain and MS. *International MS Journal, 10*(1), 14–19.

Sosnoff, J.J., & Newell, K.M. (2006). Are age-related increases in force variability due to decrements in strength? *Experimental Brain Research, 174*(1), 86-94.

Sperling, R.A., Guttmann, C.R., Hohol, M.J., Warfield, S.K., Jakab, M., Parente, M., ... Weiner, H.L. (2001). Regional magnetic resonance imaging lesion burden and cognitive function in multiple sclerosis. A longitudinal study. *Archives of Neurology, 58*(1), 115-121.

Stam, C.J., Jones, B.F., Manshanden, I., van Cappellen van Walsum, A.M., Montez, T., Verbunt, J.P., ... Scheltens, P. (2006). Magnetoencephalographic evaluation of resting-state functional connectivity in Alzheimer's disease. *NeuroImage, 32*(3), 1335–1344.

Starr, J.M., Leaper, S.A., Murray, A.D., Lemmon, H.A., Staff, R.T., Deary, I.J., & Whalley, L.J. (2003). Brain white matter lesions detected by magnetic resonance imaging are associated with balance and gait speed. *Journal of Neurology Neurosurgery & Psychiatry. 74*(1):94-98.

Stebbins, G.T., Nyenhuis, D.L., Wang, C., Cox, J.L., Freels, S., Bangen, K., ... Gorelick, P.B. (2008). Gray matter atrophy in patients with ischemic stroke with cognitive impairment. *Stroke, 39*(3), 785-793.

Steinberg, M., Leoutsakos, J-M,S., Podewils, L.J., & Lyketsos, C.G. (2009). Evaluation of a home-based exercise program in the treatment of Alzheimer's disease: The maximizing independence in dementia (MIND) study. International Journal of Geriatric Psychiatry, 24(7), 680-685.

Stephens, S., Kenny, R.A., Rowan, E., Kalaria, R.N., Bradbury, M., Pearce, R., ... Ballard, C.G. (2005). Association between mild vascular cognitive impairment and impaired activities of daily living in older stroke survivors without dementia. *Journal of the American Geriatrics Society, 53*(1), 103-107.

Stern, Y., Moeller, J.R., Anderson, K.E., Luber, B., Zubin, N.R., DiMauro, A.A., ... Sackeim, H.A. (2000). Different brain networks mediate task performance in normal aging and AD. *Neurology, 55*(9), 1291-1297.

Stevens, J.C. (1992). Aging and spatial acuity of touch. *Journals of Gerontology, 47*(1), P35-P40.

Stewart, K.J. (2002). Exercise training and the cardiovascular consequences of type 2 diabetes and hypertension. *Journal of the American Medical Assocation, 288*(13), 1622-1631.

Stolze, H., Klebe, S., Petersen, G., Raethjen, J., Wenzelburger, R., Witt, K., & Deuschl, G. (2002). Typical features of cerebellar ataxic gait. *Journal of Neurology, Neurosurgery & Psychiatry, 73*(3), 310-312.

Strenk, S.A., Semmlow, J.L., Strenk, L.M., Munoz, P., Gronlund-Jacob, J., & DeMarco, J.K. (1999). Age-related changes in human ciliary muscle and lens: A magnetic resonance imaging study. *Investigative Ophthalmology & Visual Science, 40*(6), 1162-1169.

Strik, W.K., Fallgatter, A.J., Brandeis, D., & Pascual-Marqui, R.D. (1998). Three-dimensional tomography of event-related potentials during response inhibition: Evidence for phasic frontal lobe activation. *Electroencephalography and Clinical Neurophysiology, 108*(4), 406-413.

Sullivan, P.G., & Brown, M.R. (2005). Mitochondrial aging and dysfunction in Alzheimer's disease. *Progress in Neuro-Psychopharmacology & Biological Psychiatry, 29*(3), 407-410.

Sultzer, D.L., Mahler, M.E., Mandelkern, M.A., Cummings, J.L., van Gorp, W.G., Hinkin, C.H., & Berisford, M.A. (1995). The relationship between psychiatric symptoms and regional cortical metabolism in Alzheimer's disease. *Journal of Neuropsychiatry and Clinical Neurosciences, 7*(4), 476-484.

Suva, D., Favre, I., Kraftsik, R., Esteban, M., Lobrinus, A., & Miklossy, J. (1999). Primary motor cortex involvement in Alzheimer disease. *Journal of Neuropathology and Experimental Neurology, 58*(11), 1125-1134.

Suzuki, M., Miyai, I., Ono, T., & Kubota, K. (2008). Activities in the frontal cortex and gait performance are modulated by preparation. An fNIRS study. *NeuroImage, 39*(2), 600-607.

Svendsen, K.B., Jensen, T.S., Overvad, K., Hansen, H.J., Koch-Henriksen, N., & Bach, F.W. (2003). Pain in patients with multiple sclerosis. A population-based study. *Archives of Neurology, 60*(8), 1089-1094.

Swaab, D.F. (1991). Brain aging and Alzheimer's disease, 'wear and tear' versus 'use it or lose it'. *Neurobiology of Aging, 12*(4), 317-324.

Swaab, D.F. (1997). Neurobiology and neuropathology of the human hypothalamus. In: F.E. Bloom, A. Björklund & T. Hökfelt (Eds.), Handbook of Chemical Neuroanatomy. The Primate Nervous System, Part I. Vol. 13 (pp. 39-137). Amsterdam: Elsevier Science.

Swaab, D.F. (2003). Nuclei of the human hypothalamus. Part 1. In: M.J. Aminoss, S. Boller & D.F. Swaab (Eds.), Handbook of Clinical Neurology, Vol. 79. Amsterdam: Elsevier Science.

Swaab, D.F. (2004). Neuropathology of the human hypothalamus and adjacent structures. Part 2. In: M.J. Aminoss, S. Boller & D.F. Swaab (Eds.), Handbook of Clinical Neurology, Vol. 80. Amsterdam: Elsevier Science.

Swaab, D.F., Hofman, M.A., Lucassen, P.J., Salehi, A., & Uylings, H.B.M. (1994). Neuronal atrophy, not cell death, is the main hallmark of Alzheimer's disease. *Neurobiology of Aging, 15*(3), 369-371.

Swaab, D.F., Lucassen, P.J., Salehi, A., Scherder, E.J.A., van Someren, E.W.J., & Verwer, R.W.H. (1998). Reduced neuronal activity and reactivation in Alzheimer's disease. In F.W. van Leeuwen, A. Salehi, R.J. Giger, A.J.G.D. Holtmaat, & J. Verhaagen (Eds.), Progress in Brain Research, Vol. 117. (pp. 343-377). Amsterdam: Elsevier Science.

Sweeney, J.A., Rosano, C., Berman, R.A., & Luna, B. (2001). Inhibitory control of attention declines more than working memory during normal aging. *Neurobiology of Aging, 22*(1), 39-47.

Talerico, K.A., & Evans, L.K. (2001). Responding to safety issues in frontotemporal dementias. *Neurology, 56*(11), S52-S55.

Tamada, T., Miyauchi, S., Imamizu, H., Yoshioka, T., & Kawato, M. (1999). Cerebro-cerebellar functional connectivity revealed by the laterality index in tool-use learning. *Neuroreport, 10*(2), 325-331.

Taoka, T., Iwasaki, S., Sakamoto, M., Nakagawa, H., Fukusumi, A., Myochin, K., ... Kichikawa, K. (2006). Diffusion anisotropy and diffusivity of white matter tracts within the temporal stem in Alzheimer disease: Evaluation of the 'tract of interest' by diffusion tensor tractography. *American Journal of Neuroradiology, 27*(5), 1040-1045.

Tariot, P.N. (1994). Alzheimer disease: An overview. *Alzheimer Disease and Associated Disorders, 8* (Suppl. 2), S4-S11.

Taylor, L.J., & Herr, K. (2003). Pain intensity assessment: a comparison of selected pain intensity scales for use in cognitively intact and cognitively impaired African American older adults. *Pain Management Nursing, 4*(2), 87-95.

Tedeschi, G., Cirillo, M., Tessitore, A., & Cirillo, S. (2008). Alzheimer's disease and other dementing conditions. *Neurological Sciences, 29*(Suppl. 3), S301-S307.

Thomas, K.M., Hunt, R.H., Vizueta, N., Sommer, T., Durston, S., Yang, Y., & Worden, M.S. (2004). Evidence of developmental differences in implicit sequence learning: An fMRI study of children and adults. *Journal of Cognitive Neuroscience, 16*(8), 1339-1351.

Thomas, V.S., & Hageman, P.A. (2003). Can neuromuscular strength and function in people with dementia be rehabilitated using resistance-exercise training? Results from a preliminary intervention study. *Journals of Gerontology Series A-Biological Sciences and Medical Sciences, 58*(8), 746-751.

Thompson, J.R., Gibson, J.M., & Jagger, C. (1989). The association between visual impairment and mortality in elderly people. *Age and Ageing, 18*(2), 83-88.

Thompson, P.D., & Nutt, J.G. (2007). Higher level gait disorders. *Journal of Neural Transmission, 114* (10), 1305-1307.

Thompson, P.M., Hayashi, K.M., Dutton, R.A., Chiang, M.C., Leow, A.D., Sowell, E.R., ... Toga, A.W. (2007). Tracking Alzheimer's disease. *Annals of the New York Academy of Sciences. 1097*, 183-214.

Tognoni, G., Ceravolo, R., Nucciarone, B., Bianchi, F., Dell'Agnello, G., Ghicopulos, I., Siciliano, G., & Murri, L. (2005). From mild cognitive impairment to dementia: A prevalence study in a district of Tuscany, Italy. *Acta Neurologica Scandinavica, 112*(2), 65-71.

Toulotte, C., Fabre, C., Dangremont, B., Lensel, G., & Thevenon, A. (2003). Effects of physical training on the physical capacity of frail, demented patients with a history of falling: A randomised controlled trial. *Age Ageing, 32*(1), 67-73.

Trabace, L., Cassano, T., Steardo, L., Pietra, C., Villetti, G., Kendrick, K.M., & Cuomo, V. (2000). Biochemical and neurobehavioral profile of CHF2819, a novel, orally active acetylcholinesterase inhibitor for Alzheimer's disease. *Journal of Pharmacology and Experimental Therapeutics, 294*(1), 187-194.

Traykov, L., Baudic, S., Raoux, N., Latour, F., Rieu, D., Smagghe, A., & Rigaud, A.S. (2005). Patterns of memory impairment and perseverative behavior discriminate early Alzheimer's disease from subcortical vascular dementia. *Journal of the Neurological Sciences, 229*(Sp. Iss. SI), 75-79.

Tremblay, F., Wong, K., Sanderson, R., & Coté, L. (2003). Tactile spatial acuity in elderly persons: Assessment with grating domes and relationship with manual dexterity. *Somatosensory & Motor Research, 20*(2), 127-132.

Trick, G.L., & Silverman, S.E. (1991). Visual sensitivity to motion: Age-related changes and deficits in senile dementia of the Alzheimer type. *Neurology, 41*(9), 1437-1440.

Tsiptsios, I., Fountoulakis, K.N., Sitzoglou, K., Papanicolaou, A., Phokas, K., Fotiou, F., & St Kaprinis, G. (2003). Clinical and neuroimaging correlates of abnormal short-latency Somatosensory Evoked Potentials in elderly vascular dementia patients: A psychophysiological exploratory study. *Annals of General Hospital Psychiatry, 2*(1), 8.

Tuokko, H., Morris, C., & Ebert, P. (2005). Mild cognitive impairment and everyday functioning in older adults. *Neurocase, 11*(1), 40-47.

Uchida. S., Suzuki, A., Kagitani, F., & Hotta, H. (2000). Effects of age on cholinergic vasodilation of cortical cerebral blood flow vessels in rats. *Neuroscience Letters, 294*(2), 109-112.

Umetsu, A., Okuda, J., Fujii, T., Tsukiura, T., Nagasaka, T., Yanagawa, I., ... Yamadori, A. (2002). Brain activation during the fist-edge-palm test: A functional MRI study. *NeuroImage, 17*(1), 385-392.

Uylings, H.B.M., & de Brabander, J.M. (2002). Neuronal changes in normal human aging and Alzheimer's disease. *Brain and Cognition, 49*(3), 268-276.

Valentijn, S.A.M., van Boxtel, M.P.J., van Hooren, S.A.H., Bosma, H., Beckers, H.J.M., Ponds, R.W.H.M., & Jolles, J. (2005). Change in sensory functioning predicts change in cognitive functioning: Results from a 6-year follow-up in the Maastricht Aging Study. *Journal of the American Geriatrics Society, 53*(3), 374-380.

Vallis, L.A., & McFadyen, B.J. (2005). Children use different anticipatory control strategies than adults to circumvent an obstacle in the travel path. *Experimental Brain Research, 167*(1), 119-127.

van Boxtel, M.P., ten Tusscher, M.P., Metsemakers, J.F., Willems, B., & Jolles, J. (2001). Visual determinants of reduced performance on the Stroop color-word test in normal aging individuals. *Journal of Clinical and Experimental Neuropsychology, 23*(5), 620-627.

van de Pol, L.A., Hensel, A., van de Flier, W.M., Visser, P.J., Pijnenburg, Y.A.L., Barkhof, F., & Scheltens, P. (2005). Hippocampal atrophy on MRI in frontotemporal lobar degeneration and Alzheimer's disease. *Journal of Neurology, Neurosurgery and Psychiatry, 77*(4), 439-442.

van de Pol, L.A., Hensel, A., van der Flier, W.M., Visser, P.J., Pijnenburg, Y.A., Barkhof, F., & Scheltens, P. (2005). Hippocampal atrophy on MRI in frontotemporal lobar degeneration and Alzheimer's disease. *Journal of Neurology Neurosurgery & Psychiatry. 77*(4), 439-442.

Van der Flier, W.M., Van Den Heuvel, D.M., Weverling-Rijnsburger, A.W., Spilt, A., Bollen, E.L., Westendorp, R.G., Middelkoop, H.A., & Van Buchem, M.A. (2002). Cognitive decline in AD and mild cognitive impairment is associated with global brain damage. *Neurology. 59*(6):874-879.

van Duijn, C.M., & Hofman, A. (1992). Risk factors for Alzheimer's disease: The EURODEM collaborative re-analysis of case-control studies. *Neuroepidemiology 11*(Suppl. 1), 106-113.

van Gelder, B.M., Tijhuis, M.A.R., Kalmijn, S., Giampaoli, S., Nissinen, A., & Kromhout, D. (2004). Physical activity in relation to cognitive decline in elderly men. The FINE study. *Neurology, 63* (12), 2316-2321.

van Halteren-van Tilborg, I.A., Scherder, & E.J., Hulstijn, W. (2007). Motor-skill learning in Alzheimer's disease: A review with an eye to the clinical practice. *Neuropsychology Review. 17(3)*, 203-212.

van Petten, C., Plante, E., Davidson, P.S.R., Kuo, T.Y., Bajuscak, L., & Glisky, E.L. (2004). Memory and executive function in older adults: Relationships with temporal and prefrontal gray matter volumes and white matter hyperintensities. *Neuropsychologia, 42*(10), 1313-1335.

van Swieten, J.C., Stevens, M., Rosso, S.M. Rizzu, P., Joosse, M., de Koning, I., & Heutink, P. (1999). Phenotypic variation in hereditary frontotemporal dementia with tau mutations. *Annals of Neurology, 46*(4), 617-626.

Varma, A.R., Adams, W., Lloyd, J.J., Carson, K.J., Snowden, J.S., Testa, H.J., & Neary, D. (2002a). Diagnostic patterns of regional atrophy on MRI and regional cerebral blood flow change on SPECT in young onset patients with Alzheimer's disease, frontotemporal dementia and vascular dementia. *Acta Neurologica Scandinavica, 105*(4), 261-269.

Varma, A.R., Laitt, R., Lloyd, J.J. Carson, K.J., Snowden, J.S., Neary, D., & Jackson, A. (2002b). Diagnostic value of high signal abnormalities on T2 weighted MRI in the differentiation of Alzheimer's, frontotemporal and vascular dementias. *Acta Neurologica Scandinavica, 105*(5), 355-364.

Varrone, A., Pappatà, S., Caracò, C., Soricelli, A., Milan, G., Quarantelli, M., ... Salvatore, M. (2002). Voxel-based comparison of rCBF SPET images in frontotemporal dementia and Alzheimer's disease highlights the involvement of different cortical networks. *European Journal of Nuclear Medicine & Molecular Imaging, 29*(11), 1447-1454.

Verbeek, H., van Rossum, E., Zwakhalen, S.M., Kempen, G.I., & Hamers, J.P. (2009). Small, homelike care environments for older people with dementia: a literature review. *International Psychogeriatrics, 21*(2), 252-264.

Vereeck, L., Wuyts, F., Truijen, S., & van de Heyning, P. (2008). Clinical assessment of balance: Normative data, and gender and age effects. *International Journal of Audiology. 47*(2), 67-75.

Verghese, J., Wang, C., Lipton, R.B., Holtzer, R., & Xue, X. (2007). Quantitative gait dysfunction and risk of cognitive decline and dementia. *Journal of Neurology, Neurosurgery & Psychiatry, 78*(9), 929-935.

Verma, S., Yao, L., Stewart, D.J., Dumont, A.S., Anderson, T.J., & McNeill, J.H. (2001). Endothelial antagonism uncovers insulin-mediated vasorelaxation in vitro and in vivo. *Hypertension, 37*(2), 328-333.

Verschueren, S.M.P., Brumagne, S., Swinnen, S., & Cordo, P.J. (2002). The effect of aging on dynamic position sense at the ankle. *Behavioural Brain Research, 136*(2), 593-603.

Vertes, R. (1991). A PHA-L analysis of ascending projections of the dorsal raphe nucleus in the rat. *The Journal of Comparative Neurology, 313*(4), 643-668.

Villain, N., Desgranges, B., Viader, F., de la Sayette, V., Mézenge, F., Landeau, B., ... Chételat, G. (2008). Relationships between hippocampal atrophy, white matter disruption, and gray matter hypometabolism in Alzheimer's disease. *Journal of Neuroscience, 28*(24), 6174-6181.

Voelcker-Rehage, C., & Alberts, J.L. (2005). Age-related changes in grasping force modulation. *Experimental Brain Research, 166*(1), 61-70.

Vogt, B.A., & Sikes, R.W. (2000). The medial pain system, cingulate cortex, and parallel processing of nociceptive information. In: E.A. Mayer & C.B. Saper (Eds.), *Progress in Brain Research. Amsterdam,* Vol. 122 (pp. 223-235). Amsterdam: Elsevier Science.

von Hofsten, C. (2004). An action perspective on motor development. *Trends in Cognitive Neurosciences, 8*(6), 266-272.

Voytko, M.L. (1996). Cognitive functions of the basal forebrain cholinergic system in monkeys: Memory or attention? *Behavioral Brain Research, 75*(1-2), 13-25.

Waite, L.M., Grayson, D.A., Piguet, O., Creasey, H., Bennett, H.P., & Broe, G.A.(2005). Gait slowing as a predictor of incident dementia: 6-year longitudinal data from the Sydney Older Persons Study. *Journal of the Neurological Sciences, 229*(Sp. Iss. SI), 89-93.

Wang, L., van Belle, G., Kukull, W.B., Larson, E.B. (2002). Predictors of functional change: a longitudinal study of nondemented people aged 65 and older. *Journal of the American Geriatrics Society. 50*(9):1525-1534.

Wang, C., Wai, Y., Kuo, B., Yeh, Y.Y., & Wang, J. (2008). Cortical control of gait in healthy humans: an fMRI study. *Journal of Neural Transmission, 115*(8), 1149-1158.

Wang, J., Eslinger, P.J., Smith, M.B., & Yang, Q.X. (2005). Functional magnetic resonance imaging study of human olfaction and normal aging. *Journal of Gerontology: Medical Sciences, 60A*(4), 510-514.

Wang, K., Liang, M., Wang, L., Tian, L., Zhang, X., Li, K., & Jiang, T. (2007). Altered functional connectivity in early Alzheimer's disease: A resting-state fMRI study. *Human Brain Mapping, 28* (10), 967-978.

Wang, P.J., Saykin, A.J., Flashman, L.A., Wishart, H.A., Rabin, L.A., Santulli, R.B., & Mamourian, A. C. (2005). Regionally specific atrophy of the corpus callosum in AD, MCI and cognitive complaints. *Neurobiology of Aging, 27*(11), 1613-1617.

Wang, R., Yang, C., Lin, K., Chen, W., Chwang, L., & Liu, H. (2004). Weight loss, nutritional status and physical activity in patients with Alzheimer's disease. *Journal of Neurology, 251*(3), 314-320.

Ward, J. (2003). Encoding and the frontal lobes: A dissociation between retrograde and anterograde memories. *Cortex, 39*(4-5), 791-812.

Warden, V., Hurley, A.C., & Volicer, L. (2003). Development and psychometric evaluation of the Pain Assessment in Advanced Dementia (PAINAD) scale. *Journal of the American Medical Directors Association, 4*(1), 9-15.

Waseem, S., & Gwinn-Hardy, K. (2001). Pain in Parkinson's disease. Common yet seldom recognized symptom is treatable. *Postgraduate Medicine, 110*(6), 33-46.

Wenk, G.L. (2003). Neuropathologic changes in Alzheimer's disease. *The Journal of Clinical Psychiatry, 64*(Suppl. 9), 7-10.

Wentzel, C., Rockwood, K., MacKnight, C., Hachinski, V., Hogan, D.B., Feldman, H., ... McDowell, I. (2001). Progression of impairment in patients with vascular cognitive impairment without dementia. *Neurology, 57*(4), 714-716.

Werber, E.A., & Rabey, J.M. (2001). The beneficial effect of cholinesterase inhibitors on patients suffering from Parkinson's disease and dementia. *Journal of Neural Transmission, 108*(11), 1319-25.

West, R.L., Crook, T.H., & Barron, K.L. (1992). Everyday memory performance across the lifespan: Effects of age and noncognitive individual differences. *Psychology and Aging, 7*(1), 72-82.

Westerterp, K.R. (2000). Daily physical activity and ageing. *Current Opinion in Clinical Nutrition and Metabolic Care, 3*(6), 485-488.

Weuve, J., Kang, J.H., Manson, J.E., Breteler, M.M., Ware. J.H., & Grodstein, F. (2004). Physical activity, including walking, and cognitive function in older women. *Journal of the American Medical Association, 292*(12), 1454-1461.

Williams, P., & Lord, S.R. (1997). Effects of group exercise on cognitive functioning and mood in older women. *Australian and New Zealand Journal of Public Health, 21*(1), 45-52.

Willis, W.D., & Westlund, K.N. (1997). Neuroanatomy of the pain system and the pathways that modulate pain. *Journal of Clinical Neurophysiology, 14*(1), 2-31.

Wilson, M.M., & Morley, J.E. (2003). Invited review: Aging and energy balance. *Journal of Applied Physiology, 95*(4), 1728-1736.